Cancer and Cancer Symptoms

CHIEFLY ARBORIVITAL TREATMENT

WITH ILLUS'

GW00712329

ROBERT T. COOPER, M.A., M.D.

Author of Papers on Arborivital Medicine (Hahnemannian Monthly, Philadelphia); The Problems of Homoeopathy Solved; Vascular Deafness; Lecturer on Diseases of the Ear, & c.

SECOND EDITION

B. JAIN PUBLISHERS (P) LTD.
• New Delhi •

Price : Rs. 20.00

Reprint Edition : 1997
© Copyright with the Publisher
Published by :
B. Jain Publishers Pvt. Ltd.
1921, Street No. 10, Chuna Mandi
Paharganj, New Delhi - 110 055 (INDIA)
Printed at :
J. J. Offset Printers
7, Wazir Pur, Delhi

ISBN 81-7021-212-X
BOOK CODE B-3481

CANCER AND CANCER SYMPTOMS

"The subject (Cancer Treatment) is a peculiarly painful one from many points of view. If the fruits of long reflexion thereon be here too plainly set forth, its importance to the public weal, the continually increasing proportions of the evil, above all the power of the vested interests which bar improvement, must be pleaded in excuse." — HERBERT SNOW, M.D., in "Cancerous and other Tumours."

PREFATORY NOTICE.

I HAVE termed the system proposed by me for the better investigation of the curative action of plant-remedies, *Arborivital*, from the fact that this curative action is an inherent property of living plants, a truth which has hitherto been entirely unacknowledged by medical scientists.

Whether the existence of such a power was suspected by Hahnemann or not it is impossible for anyone to say, but certain it is that he considered single drops of plant remedies too strong for use when symptomatically related to disease. That these single drops—the unit or arborivital doses—are not too strong for use in malignant diseases, is amply shown in the body of this little work.

In fact, it is not possible to urge any reasonable objection to the use of these doses in suitable cases.

There is, then, obviously, no intention of initiating a new system of medicine ; between the idea conveyed by this term and a system for the better prosecution of research into the actions of a limited group of remedial agents upon a defined class of diseases, a very wide distinction must be drawn.

Confessedly the outcome and development of Hahnemann's ideas, my researches have been in no way directed to the furtherance or sustainment of existing systems of medicine.

All I lay claim to is an honest and practical inquiry into the curative actions of certain remedial agents upon what were hitherto supposed to be incurable diseases, and with the results I am proud to admit myself fully satisfied.

My position will perhaps be better understood, even at the risk of subsequent repetition, by a reference to the following letters called forth by an Editorial Article and subsequent correspondence in *Invention* newspaper :—

(*Reprinted from " Invention " of November* 5, 1898.)

"ARBORIVITAL MEDICINE."
TO THE EDITOR OF "INVENTION."

SIR,—To attempt to reply to each of your correspondents would be to trespass too greatly upon your space and upon my own time. It will suffice to point out the requirements of modern medicine and then your readers can judge if I have fulfilled these requirements.

Modern medicine has not succeeded in, and therefore requires, beyond all else, the power to remove settled disease from the human body. By settled disease I mean disease the tendency of which is to linger in the body, in fact, chronic disease, which, broadly speaking, goes on to undermine the whole system, and brings about a death of the tissues. That it is impossible to get rid of chronic disease by the ordinary means at our disposal it would be easy to show did time and space permit. What is not required, this being brought to a fair state of perfection, is an ability to conduct acute or inflammatory disease to a successful termination, the natural tendency of which form of disease being, speaking broadly, towards recovery. Now, this being the position, the question is, Are we to look to the laboratory of the chemist or to the laboratory of Nature for the dispersal of such forms of disease?

Without arguing the matter, I wish to say that I go

direct to Nature and in natural forces I obtain my remedies. A friend, who read to me the correspondence in
your issue of October 22, asked, How on earth I could
reply to all the objections? Very simply, I replied; by
appealing to very ordinary and trite facts. There happened
to be near us a plant of Begonia in a flower pot. I pointed
to this plant as being evidence to me of a *force*, and a very
powerful force. Look, I said, at its leaves and its stalks,
and observe the beauty of their formation and of the
colouration of its different parts. This plant has come
from a seed, or, if you will, a germ, which has been placed
amidst favourable surroundings—in suitable soil. *The
effect of the power of the germ depended upon the conditions
under which it was placed.* This cannot be gainsaid.
Now, I said, turn from Mother Earth to your own body.
Suppose you have a large tumour. This has come from a
germ favourably placed for development in your body; it,
like the plant, represents the result of a growth—force.

Now, if I take a living particle of the plant and throw
it into your body, it will simply depend upon the conditions as to whether that particle will manifest independent
growth or not, and the evidence of its doing so will be
from the modification or dispersal of the growth—the
tumour—already existing. To say that the particle I
throw into your body could not have such an effect is just
as absurd as to say that the particle the gardener had
placed in the soil could not result in a Begonia plant;

we know only by observing it, that the germ or seed so placed can result in a Begonia. If this line of thought be carried out, the possibility of removing disease—chronic and settled disease—cannot be questioned. It is for me to determine whether I am sufficiently conversant with the conditions under which my germ or seed will start into growth, and this, with all deference to your readers, I must be the judge of for myself. What, then, I set myself originally to do was not to kill germs, but to evolve from a study of the laws of life a more direct and efficient method of coping with chronic disease.

Should any of your readers wish for further information I will be very pleased to send them a copy of my "Problems of Homœopathy Solved." As to the practical working of the system they can write, enclosing postage, to Mr. Murrell, Elm Lodge, Feltham, Middlesex, who three months ago was supposed to be dying, after having been operated upon in the Cancer Hospital.

I am, &c.,

ROBERT T. COOPER, M.A., M.D.

November 1, 1898.

(*Reprinted from "Invention" of December* 3, 1898.)

———

"ARBORIVITAL MEDICINE."
TO THE EDITOR OF "INVENTION."

SIR,—Your correspondent, Mr. Tatham, honours me by accepting my statement that the *desideratum* in medicine is the efficient dispersal of chronic disease.

This is so unquestionable that, as he says, it " requires no comment." But as if to belie the cause of his satisfaction, he proceeds to rate me on having left the germ theory " severely alone." Considering that the germ theory has not furnished us with a satisfactory treatment of chronic disease, I am at a loss to understand what it has to do with the question ; had he read my letter carefully he would have seen that I expressly considered it outside the range of present discussion.

Mr. Tatham assumes that I consider that if one form of germ deposited amidst one set of surroundings leads to a certain result, a wholly diverse form of germ deposited in other environments must necessarily induce a morphologically similar result, or, as he expresses it, " that the projection of a living particle (of a Begonia plant) into one's body will cause the growth of a Begonia " ! This certainly is not complimentary to my observations upon germs.

Mr. Tatham, like some of your correspondents, seems

to suppose that any improvement in the treatment of chronic disease must come in exactly the way he expects. I would ask you, Sir, as Editor of *Invention*, did you ever know any great improvement to be effected by a blind subservience to prevailing methods of thought ? The very idea of such a thing is absurd.

If improvement is to be brought about in medicine as in other branches of knowledge, we must diverge from the beaten tracks, the probability being that the truth is to be found in unexpected directions.

But not only is any divergence from ordinary views likely to meet with opposition, owing to the preconceived opinions of mankind, but it has to encounter a much more serious opposition should it at all run counter to existing commercial interests.

How strong are established interests will be apparent when I state that there is no professional medical journal in the kingdom that will admit a report of a case of mine if treated with a single dose, no matter how successful the result. One journal, the *Homœopathic World*, certainly does, but this is partly a popular issue.

Even the *Monthly Homœopathic Review*, to which I contributed frequently for some twenty-five years, will not now admit a case from me if cured with a single drop of a plant remedy, although quite ready to insert one if treated with successive doses of a millionth part of the same drop ! This is delightful on the part of a profession that penalises secrecy by expulsion! They refuse to publish your facts if at all disagreeable, and unfrock you if you keep back information.

That the treatment of chronic disease by single doses of medicine is no new thing, it would be easy to show; and the absolute necessity for using such in certain obstinate cases has been insisted upon by Hahnemann and all his really prominent followers, past and present, without, I think, a single exception. Among the former I may name Doctors Curie, John Epps, David Wilson, the late Doctor Hilbers, of Brighton; Constantine Hering, Jahr, &c., and amongst the latter are to be counted the foremost homœopathic doctors in London, Dr. Compton Burnett, of Wimpole Street, W., and Finsbury Circus; Dr. J. H. Clarke, of Clarges Street, Piccadilly, and of Cornhill; Dr. Skinner Dr. Berridge, and many others.

In fact, the prejudices of mankind are so strong in favour of continuous dosing in every kind of case that it has been found necessary to give unmedicated doses in between the really active ones. The fact, therefore, is, that thousands of patients have been treated by single doses without their knowing it! Whether it is more exalted to keep the public in ignorance of the real situation, or to explain the truth to them and to *prove* it, I leave your readers to judge. One thing is perfectly certain, if the homœopaths think they can suppress the truth in an age of enlightenment like this they are grievously mistaken. That

Hahnemann considered the single dose an essential part of his system and that he did not seek to comprehend it, is evident from this footnote to pp. 155-6 of vol. i. of his "Chronic Diseases," published at New York, 1845 :—"My doctrines," says Hahnemann in regard to the magnitude and repetition of the doses, " will be doubted for years, even by the greater number of homœopathic physicians." And he goes on : " My proposition, however, is not one of those which ought to be comprehended, nor one which ought to be blindly believed. No one is bound either to comprehend or to believe that proposition : I (Hahnemann) do not comprehend it, but the facts speak for themselves." The proposition here referred to was that the carefully selected remedy should act until it had completed its effect, and that doses should be able to influence inveterate disease for two or three, or even for forty or fifty days.

What I profess to have done is to give a reasonable explanation that leads to a comprehension of this admitted fact, and to confine myself to what Hahnemann and many of his followers considered too strong a dose, namely, a single drop of plant juice.

But all this theory sinks into insignificance compared with practical experience. Your correspondent, Mr. Tatham, while so solicitous as to the truth, did not take the trouble to investigate the case I presented to your readers—that of a growth that had been operated on in the Cancer Hospital at Brompton.

Not to weary your readers, I will submit (1) a copy of the certificate of the doctor attending the patient after removal from the Cancer Hospital, and (2) a copy of the patient's letter to me subsequently to leaving Shepherd's Bush. Attention to the dates is important, bearing in mind that I first saw this patient July 22, and that not until July 28 was he placed on single doses.

(1)   " July 19, 1898.

" This is to certify that Mr. George A. Murrell, of 33, Richmond Road, Shepherd's Bush, has been under my care for the last six months, suffering from a tumour near the pyloric end of the stomach, and is totally unable to follow any employment.

(Signed)   " M.D., M.R.C.S., L.R.C.P."
(Name omitted for obvious reasons.)

(2)   " Elm Lodge, Feltham, Middlesex,
                                    "October 14, 1898.

" Dr. Cooper,

" DEAR SIR,—I am pleased to tell you that your medicine has had the desired effect. I feel nothing fresh from the old complaint except that I am still a bit weak. My appetite is wonderfully good, in fact, I cannot get enough to eat. I hope it will continue so, as I shall then soon get strong again and be able to do something I am anxious to do. The only thing I fear is the winter, otherwise I have never been so well for nearly twenty years. I get no pains after food like I used to do, nor do I suffer from indigestion in any way, everything seems to agree with me and I feel always hungry. I do not vomit, and sleep fairly well at night. Again thanking you for your kindness, with best wishes,

"I am, dear Sir, very faithfully yours,
"GEORGE A. MURRELL."

If this does not establish my position nothing will.

Yours, &c.,

ROBERT T. COOPER, M.A., M.D.

November 29, 1898.

The preparations of remedies used are tinctures made on the spot from living plants, proof spirit being employed for the sake of preserving their inherent properties.

Some of my tinctures (none of those used in this work) are made by allowing the spirit to come into contact with the living plant—the branch, while still attached, being kept plunged in the spirit and exposed to sunlight while thus immersed—*heliosthened*, as I term it.

How obvious it is that our present fiscal system is

inimical to the progress of medical science, is evident when we reflect that the success of beer and of medicine is judged of largely by the same standard—the amount consumed and the accruing gain; hence I cannot anticipate any very favourable reception in some quarters for this new departure.

In the higher spheres of thought—such as the physician's ought to be—I do certainly anticipate for it a favourable reception; the physician's sole consideration ought to be the conquest of disease, nor is it worth while, in this short life of ours, to have any other object in view.

It is quite true that there has not been discovered by myself or by any authority a specific for all varieties of cancer, or for that matter for all varieties of any other form of disease. But what is true of other diseases is, I maintain, true of cancer, and this is that each case should be singled out and should constitute a special study, with a view not merely for the ascertainment of its nomenclature, but more a great deal for the selection of the indicated remedy; for while it is evident that there is not one specific for all kinds of cancer, it is equally true there are many specifics for the numerous varieties of malignant disease.

I am quite aware that in the cases narrated the indications relied upon for prescribing certain remedies may appear to be insufficient, but where much must necessarily be instinctive and insufficiently proved, it is better to defer explanations till the reasons for selection are less doubtful and more capable of explanation.

That every remedy which is accepted as curative of a given disease must be proved to be able to produce a disease that is alike to it in every particular, is simply obstructive nonsense. Obstructive, because no remedies have ever produced natural diseases.

Remedial agents do undoubtedly produce symptoms like to those present in all diseases, and that such symptoms constitute signatures or sign-boards by which the prescription of remedies can be rendered more

2

accurate and infinitely more successful, is unquestionable.

The attempt must fail to find a drug the properties and pathogenetic quantity of which are, in each case, proved to correspond with the disease present; for it is nowadays maintained that not alone must the symptoms produced on the healthy by the drug correspond with those of the disease to be treated, but the dose in which it is capable of affecting the healthy must be the dose required in disease. This leads us to allopathic dosage with a vengeance, and is in every way inconsistent with facts.

The attempt to ignore all properties in drugs that have not been proved by the establishment of a coarse pathological change, is to unduly limit our remedial measures; the production of symptoms alone gives us unerring indications, if these are characteristic of the disease to be treated.

In cancer cases, as in all other cases, symptoms must

be our principal guide ; success in treatment will depend upon the repetition of the remedy almost as much as upon its choice. This is one of the great teachings of this work.

18, *Wimpole Street, W.*

CONTENTS.

Chapter I.

Contents

CHAPTER IV.

CHAPTER V.

CHAPTER VI.

Chapter VII.

Chapter VIII.

CANCER AND CANCER SYMPTOMS.

CHAPTER I.

Arborivital Medicine: its meaning.—The necessity for investigating action of Single Doses.—Remedies act over a long period of time.—Special preparations of plant-remedies not absolutely necessary.—Medical Education not in accordance with Nature.— The Cancers easily acted on; explanation.—Illustrative Case.— Cancer contrasted with Chronic Deafness and other Chronic Diseases.—Case of Hodgkin's Disease: lessons to be learned from it.

IN a series of papers published in the *Hahnemannian Monthly* of Philadelphia, I sketched out a system for the better investigation of medicinal substances, and particularly of plant-remedies, to which I gave the name Arborivital Medicine.

The idea underlying the proposal is, that if it is required to discover the actions of plant-remedies and their in-

I

fluence upon chronic forms of disease, it is absolutely necessary that we start *de novo*, and investigate the actions not alone of single remedies, as Hahnemann had done, but still more of single doses of these remedies; and I further set out that in investigating the effects of these single doses I had found that there existed in plant-remedies a force which Hahnemann had strangely left unacknowledged, and which acted by virtue of a power in all respects similar to a germinating power in the human body.

Hahnemann, it is well known, claimed for his special preparations of remedies—mineral as well as vegetable substances—a property of lingering in the human body and continuing to act for a much longer time than had previously been suspected. Such a power he claimed for his dilutions and triturations, but he did not claim, or if he did, none of his followers have since his time claimed, that substances possess any such power apart from these artificial preparations.

Hahnemann's own wording on the subject is, I admit, not very clear, and a lengthy discussion on the subject would be undesirable.

My contention, in a word, is this, that in the living plants we get a force which, if applied in accordance with the laws of Life to disease, will arrest its progress, and even cause its dispersal. Further, that while artificial preparations, dilutions, and triturations are required for the better demonstration of such a force in mineral substances, they are not required for proving the existence of a like force in plant-remedies. To this force I gave the name arborivital, and the action that results therefrom Arborivital Action.

I do not hesitate to affirm that the whole state of medical education is in every way unnatural, and that this accounts for the fact that little or nothing is known of the actions of our commonest plants by men supposed to be our foremost medical practitioners; and I further state that some of the most easily acted upon forms of chronic disease, such as are the cancers, have for this reason remained, at this enlightened age, upon the list of uncured and incurable diseases.[1]

---

[1] The curriculum of education adopted for the practitioner of medicine is more absurd than the public imagines.

In former days the young student had some chance of familiarising himself at starting with the practical work of his profession, for he became an apprentice or assistant to an experienced practitioner and had an opportunity of seeing what were the every day duties of a working member of the craft.

Now this is all changed; the student is debarred by the Medical Council from doing any kind of work until he is qualified.

In order to be qualified he has to keep studying anatomy and materia medica for two years before he is allowed to feel a pulse, look at a tongue, or give a dose of medicine.

At the end of these two years, and before he has yet looked at a patient, he is examined in what ?—in materia medica : in other words, in the actions and doses of medicines.

Doses did I say ? yes, the doses, *i.e.*, the largest amount of *medicine* that can be given short of poisoning the patient.

If the diligent youngster dares to suggest anything above or below this standard, he is forthwith relegated to his studies ; to the enrichment of the Conjoint Board, and the abolition in himself of all sense of the fitness of things.

Nothing is more common than to hear old and experienced medical men aver that they do not believe in the actions of medicines.

A still worse fate, however, attends the aspirant to a knowledge of Homœopathy. Having devoted five or six years of the best portion of the thirty years of his probable professional life to an indoctrination into the mysteries of allopathy and having been declared by august qualifying bodies to be endowed with knowledge sufficient to deal with the responsibilities necessarily attendant upon the treatment of disease, not a single case of which he has ever treated, he can then, but not till then, avail himself of private judgment and make inquiry into advanced medicine.

Here, however, any little pride he might feel in having successfully acquitted himself, so far, in his professional career, is destined to receive a rude shock.

No sooner does he enter as a student at the London Homœopathic Hospital, than the information is vouchsafed him that within these sacred precincts, no tongue must be looked at, or pulse felt by any other than a Member of the British Homœopathic Society ; belief must come before conviction and must rest upon the evidence of things not seen. And this is the method adopted by a reforming body to secure the enlightenment of the coming generation in the system of Hahnemann. Our special wonder may well be excited at such things as these !

Considering that these very men have been filling the systems of suffering human beings all their lives with medicines, it is rather too much of an absurdity.

If these same medical men had been put on to investigate the actions of our common plants, and restricted in their prescriptions to single doses and to chronic and non-urgent cases of disease, I do not hesitate to say they would either, and rightly so, have been in the early days of their career stopped from proceeding further, or would have given evidence of their fitness for their profession by making valuable observations. The real fact is that the investigation of our plant-remedies is extremely simple and free from risk, if we but confine ourselves to single doses and to chronic forms of disease.

Moreover, it is also a fact that the most easily acted upon of all forms of chronic disease are, as just hinted at, the tumours, especially internal ones, whether cancerous or otherwise. It is the object of this pamphlet to support these last two propositions.

Before going further let me illustrate this assertion that the internal cancerous tumours can be easily acted on.

A lady asked me if I would take up the case of a poor woman suffering from cancer, in whom the right kidney had been removed some eighteen months before, and in whom the cancer had broken out again at the site of the operation and around the bladder.

Without seeing the patient, and from my experience in such cases, I replied that in all probability there was a great deal of cancerous growth present, and that if so, the likelihood was in favour of its being easily acted on, and consequently, that the disease would give out almost immediately she took a dose of the indicated remedy. The patient, therefore, I went on to say, will probably be frightened, and discontinue treatment.

The lady's reply was significant: "There is not the slightest fear of the poor woman being frightened, for she is now under the influence of morphia, and is entirely despaired of by all the doctors who have seen her." On

February, 10, 1899, I sent her a dose of a very simple remedy the saffron crocus—and on the 14th her daughter came to me to know what was to be done, as her mother, though constipated previously, had next day after the dose, broken out into the most violent diarrhœa; even her food passed through her at once, and she felt fearfully depressed and low.

Recognising the fact that all this was to be fully explained by the out-pouring of the disease, I simply advised copious draughts of very hot water in sips, and the discontinuance as far as possible of the morphia she had been taking.

It is such evidence as this in numbers of cases that entirely justifies me in saying that the internal cancers admit of more satisfactory proof of being acted upon by internal medication than any forms of chronic disease. Take, for example, a chronic deafness—vascular deafness,[1]

---

[1] The terms applied by the Author to the most usual form of Chronic Deafness, the initial lesion of which is a diffused vasculitis

or a chronic psoriasis, or long-lasting skin affection, it is not possible in any varieties of these affections to demonstrate so satisfactorily to either patient or doctor that the internal medicine is in operation, as was done in the above instance.

In all varieties of chronic disease the same *force* may be thrown into the system, and may begin working from the first, yet the evidence of its activity is at once apparent in the cancers, and it may not be demonstrable in the others for weeks, or even months. And is this unreasonable? In such a condition as cancerous tumours we get myriads of germs accumulated in one part of the body, the inference being that Nature, always conservative, protects and prolongs the life of the individual by causing these germs to collect in one region, rather than allow the poisonous influence to have full sway by their

---

and the consequence, the thickening and stiffening of the Mucous Membrane (of Toynbee), or the Proliferous Catarrh (of Roosa). *Vide* "Vascular Deafness," Baillière, Tindall and Cox, London, 1886.

3

dissemination throughout the various structures of the human body.

If this be the case, the effect of the indicated remedy will be proportionate to the size of the accumulated mass and the ease with which it can be acted on.

If, then, the ignorant and superstitious idea obtains that there must be some proportion between the amount of disease material and the size and virulence of the dispersing agent, any attempt at curing the disease is simply hopeless. For is it not evident that if a large quantity of such a substance is necessarily associated with a proportionate amount of force, such force, if in relationship with the disease, will be so great as to cause a rapid giving way of diseased tissue and will thus tend to poison the patient?

While if, in such a case as the above, the doses, though small are too frequently repeated, the effect will be the same, and the too rapid dispersal of the diseased material will act as a poison not alone to the life of the adjoining issues but to that of the patient thus rapidly infected?

That medicines—simple plant-remedies—can thus influence these forms of disease is not a matter of mere theory; my knowledge of it is evolved from deliberate clinical observation extending over more than thirty years. The matter is simply one of relationship, it is not a matter of quantity of material.

The seed of a globe turnip (*Brassica Rapa*) is said to multiply its bulk in the ground seventeen million of times, the resulting effect being in no way due to the size of the original seed but to the relationship that exists between the soil and the germ or seed placed there.

In the case of cancer referred to, the evidence is almost as strong in favour of an action resulting from the dose, as it is that the turnip resulted from the originating seed. The power is manifest, it is strong, and science having obtained such a power ought to find means to make it efficient—efficient, that is, for curative purposes.

Were there no evidence forthcoming but that furnished by the above case, it alone would prove the preliminary statement that the cancers, and especially the internal ones, can easily be acted on.

But can this Force, so powerful in disturbing a disease mass, be utilised for curative purposes? In the case referred to, an immense carcinomatous mass extended from close below the liver down to the pelvis of the right side, and at the site of operation this pointed and threatened to ulcerate. A patient whose body is so full of cancerous material, and with but a single kidney left after the operator has done his work, is not under any circumstances likely to recover; but that she is being acted upon, and acted upon beneficially, is evident from the pains having changed in character and severity—from stabbing, shooting pains to dull and dragging ones—and from the fact that the patient no longer requires morphia for her pains, and is having sufficient sleep. Though, as I write, a fortnight has elapsed since this patient took a dose of a very simple remedy, Juniper comm., given in consequence of the Polyuria that existed before the cancer was detected, her entreaty is not to be given another yet awhile; and she is perfectly right. The action started is a beneficial one, but it is attended with greater changes than the poor patient can comfortably endure. Its violence must be allowed to tone down before a repetition of such effects can be safely endured.

The subsequent course of the disease was characteristic. The patient went on very well and free from pain until on 3rd September I gave her a dose of silphium perfoliatum. At the time of taking it she had been getting on very fairly, the swelling, which had threatened to press up dangerously against the chest, had lessened; and the condition might have been regarded as one of remarkable quiescence, no change taking place either way.

Immediately after the dose a gnawing pain in the swelling set in and the bowels became confined, and the scar left by the eviscerated kidney began irritating and in four or five days discharge was noticed. This discharge continued to increase till a large opening formed, from which a profuse clear fluid went on pouring away night and day, from the end of September to 11th December following. On the night of 10th December she was so free from pain and suffering that her daughter, who had attended her assiduously all through, left with every expectation that her mother's rest would be undisturbed. However, in the early morning (about 2 a.m.) sinking set in, and in about an hour she passed away peaceably and happily and without a particle of pain.

What is the meaning of all this? The meaning of it is, that the vital powers had become exhausted by the draining away of the disease, an out-pouring having been effected by the unit dose of silphium given 3rd September. This out-pouring would have been *curative* had the amount of cancerous material been less in quantity; that it was undoubtedly *natural*, is proved by the absence of pain, the shrinkage of the cancerous mass, which was very obvious, and the general improvement in the patient's condition during its continuance. In other words, the evidence in favour of there being in operation a form of activity other than the activity of the cancer force itself, subsequently to the exhibition of the indicated remedy, is as conclusive as anything can be in such matters.

That heaped up disease, in the form of a cancerous mass, can be set free by the action of remedies, is placed, in my opinion, almost beyond dispute by the case of a lady, aged 54, the left side of whose neck was one great mass of cancerous glands—a truly malignant form of Hodgkin's disease. Three months before seeing me this patient had presented herself at Charing Cross Hospital, where her case was very properly declared hopeless, and an operation refused. In the meantime the disease had much extended, and when I saw her, masses of cancerous material existed on the right side of nape of neck, as well as those on the side and below the collar bone on the left. On January 5 I prescribed a unit dose and an ointment of scrophul. nodosa, and on the 19th following had in a report that a diffused rash, looking like that of measles, had spread over the body and face immediately after taking my medicine, and that otherwise she had improved ; the phlegm coming up in the throat was less and the bowels were more regular.   Ruta graveolens in unit dose and ointment was then given, and on February 2 following, she was reported as feeling much better and could swallow better.   The swellings, though the same in size, had become tender to the touch.

Now, my inference from all this was that the patient had been strongly acted upon, as shown in the first interval by this "measles" eruption, and in the second interval by the tenderness of the swellings, and throughout both intervals by the general improvement in the patient's feelings.   My advice, therefore, was to absolutely discontinue all medicines, as I felt sure a force was acting upon the swellings, and that she ran the risk of having the disease set free too quickly.   This was proved to my mind most unmistakably by the subsequent progress.

On February 14 report came in that for three days

there had been great difficulty in breathing and in swallowing, and to this my reply was that I could not sanction the giving of ordinary remedies, and that the patient was simply to sip constantly of lemon juice and hot water.

In about three weeks afterwards I was forwarded, by two messengers well acquainted with the deceased, a flurried letter, written by her daughter, to the effect that they had left the patient only too long without medicine, and that by the time a doctor was called in mortification had set in, and that the poor patient had died that morning. It was obvious from the tone of the letter that a rival practitioner had been making disparaging remarks, as sometimes happens. But this did not prevent my putting some questions to the bearers of this unhappy intelligence.

Firstly I asked, " Did the patient die in pain ? " Reply, " Oh no! not in the least." " And where, may I ask was the mortification ? " Reply, " Across the loins; the parts turned quite black before she died." "And what became of the swellings ? " Reply, "Oh, they went entirely away; there was not a vestige to be seen of them before she died." "Well, then," I said, "can you not see what took place? The medicines acted on the disease and acted beneficially, but the diseased material being in such large quantity, and discharging itself as it did through the system, an undue amount of poison was thrown upon the chief emunctories, the kidneys, and these, unable to bear the strain, mortified, together with the adjoining structures, hence the blackened appearance of the loins. This only shows the extreme naturalness of the process in operation, the patient going out of the world in a condition perfectly painless and in her senses, not in terrific agony, only subduable by obliteration of sensation by morphia."

Let, then, there be no mistake about the pronouncement made. Cancer-tissue, when accumulated in any one part of the body, can, generally speaking, be easily acted upon, much more easily than even a fatty tumour or a tuberculous mass ; the effect of remedies ought to be carefully watched, so as to prevent a too rapid dislodgment of the disease ; under any circumstances there is great danger to the patient's life if the cancer mass be large, by the too rapid outpouring of the cancer poison ; nothing contributes to this rapidity of flow so much as the constant repetition of remedies ; and, therefore, by far the safest plan is to allow a single dose to expend itself upon the disease, and to be careful not to interpose even such apparently harmless things as ointments, lest the effect upon the disease should be too great.

Of course, these remarks apply to remedies indicated by reason of their symptomatic relationship to the disease, and to forms of the disease that are in a fairly plastic condition, and not like some osteoid cancers inactive and unyielding.

CHAPTER II.

—

THE matter, then, is one of sympathetic relationship: the life of a collection of cancer cells obeys the same laws as the life of any other living body. It has come into being by a process of germination and it is to be dispersed by a force that sets agoing a similar but antagonising process. The difficulty of cure lies in the difficulty in discovering the sympathetic force.

But just as the experienced gardener knows the conditions that are most favourable for development of the energies of certain seeds, so ought the experienced practitioner to know the conditions that in the diseased patient will call into activity the curative energies of his remedy.

The consideration of this aspect of the question is likely to lead to much that is controverted ; it will suffice to say that I have met with very little difficulty in this particular class of diseases in arriving at the indicated remedies.

In this regard I have not allowed myself to be swayed by the teachings of the high dilutionists of the Homœopathic School, or by the teachings of those who contend that some special symptom should constitute a key-note and that this should be our guide to the selection of the remedy ; nor have I been guided by the more modern and material school, who insist that the curative dose should correspond in size with the pathogenic dose, and that no remedy can be relied on as a curative unless it has produced the actual disease for which it is prescribed.

On the contrary, I take into consideration all the

bearings both of the disease tendencies and of the symptoms past and present, and in accordance with these I select my remedy.

Thus, in the case of abdominal cancer referred to, I learned before prescribing that the period came dark and in clotted lumps, that she had had a sensation of something moving inside the abdomen, with a livid complexion changing now and then to yellow, and a general feeling of pressure in the abdomen, with weighty feeling towards the womb; these, added to my general experience with the effects of this particular remedy, led me to Crocus Sativus.

But it is impossible to dwell on such particulars for very long; they would by themselves fill a volume.

The physician prescribing for such cases as these may well be compared with the experienced gardener who bases his selection of the suitable soil for particular seeds upon a general experience, much of which it is impossible to communicate by word of mouth.

It is easy for the gardener to state the plain fact of having chosen a particular soil and a special season for any given seed, but he can do little more than this; he has probably forgotten the many little experiences that from time to time influenced him—it may be unconsciously—in his determination. His advantage over the doctor largely resides in the fact that from boyhood he has been in the habit of gardening; the doctor has never prescribed until he theoretically knew much, and practically knew nothing; until, in fact, the best part of his life was lost in acquiring the crudest theories of the actions of medicines.

To go on to actual experience. Take this case of CANCER OF THE PYLORUS   Geo. A. Murrell, aged 40, first seen by me July 22, 1898.

History.—Fifteen or eighteen years subject to dyspeptic pains, and twelve years ago strained himself lifting a kitchen range; felt the strain severely below the chest, and dates his suffering from then, though even before this was dyspeptic. Was treated in the Heart Hospital under

Dr. ——, after having been an out-patient for six months previously. Here his heart was pronounced affected, with old pleuritic sounds down left side, along with ulceration of the stomach. Then as out-patient (he was discharged from Hospital end of October, 1896) was again treated, chiefly with electricity.

In the middle of January, 1898, severe pains set in between the liver and stomach and he went into Westminster Hospital, the diagnosis being neuralgia of the stomach from gastric catarrh. Was discharged unrelieved ; and was then seen by several other physieians, and in March was advised to go into the Cancer Hospital, Brompton, where he was operated on ; the statement made to him after the operation being that adhesions had been found between the stomach and thoracic wall, with a cancerous growth and thickening of the pyloric extremity of the duodenum, and that it was impossible to remove all the diseased tissue. Some temporary relief followed upon the operation, and he was discharged from the hospital under promise of his returning if pain reappeared.

The patient from whom these particulars are gathered, writes to me that " The Cancer Hospital also arranged with Dr. D——, a French specialist, to come over (to the Hospital) and I (the patient) consented to another operation under him ; but when my case was fully explained to him he went back (to France) without doing anything, as I understood he could not do me any good."

This was after having obtained re-admission to the hospital owing to the return of his agonising pains. After being six weeks in hospital on this second occasion he returned home, and was assured by his own doctor that everything possible had been done for him, and that he could not possibly live long, and that he must bear the pain while life lasted.

The copy of his doctor's certificate is in my possession, dated July 19, in which it is stated that the patient " is totally unable to follow any employment."[1]

---

[1] Referred to in the Prefatory Notice.

The case, therefore, admits of no doubt as to its nature or as to its severity.

I first saw him on the evening of July 22, 1898 ; he was then writhing in agony on his bed, and could keep nothing long on his stomach ; warm foods relieved, cold drinks aggravated.

The pains were worse at night, and began in the stomach, spreading from there to the heart and between the shoulders, as if an iron brick were being forced through the stomach and chest.

The patient felt the growth to be rapidly enlarging, and pointed to the visible bulging underneath the attachment of the diaphragm, where there is marked dulness on percussion, the bulging extending to scrobiculus cordis. His tongue is red and coated towards the back, bowels confined, though sometimes has diarrhœa.

His family history is good, except that his father died at the age of 73 of gastric ulceration.

On July 27 he wrote that he had had terrible pains on

Saturday the 23rd, and had vomited twice; at 6 o'clock, p.m. of this day had taken a unit dose of Ornithogalum Umbellatum, and afterwards reported that it was followed by great pains, he felt almost frantic at 3 a.m. and again at 1 p.m., when the bowels acted. At 3 a.m. he began taking 3 grains every third hour of Carbo Vegetabilis 3x. The pain, however, still kept on, and affected not alone the stomach but the whole body, and as he thought the Carbo increased the pains he left it off on the Tuesday following. On the next day he wrote me that since being under me a frothy substance comes up which gives great relief.

From this report I concluded the Ornithogalum Umbel. had touched the disease, and had acted beneficially, though restricted in its operation by the Carbo Vegetabilis. The expulsion of a frothy substance with relief was, I considered, sufficient evidence of beneficial action. For this reason I sent him Ornithogalum Umbel. again, and in unit dose. This he took on the evening of July 28, and almost immediately after began bringing up a black jelly-like substance, with great relief to pain and a general improvement in his condition. Being away from town in August the patient frequently wrote me, the report on August 29 being as follows :—" I am pleased to tell you that I still keep fairly well, although at times I have great pain in the lower part of the stomach. I have also great difficulty in going to sleep, owing to the creepy sensation in my limbs. I also find that when I sit down my legs and feet go all of a creep, and I am unable to keep still, and cannot read unless I walk about. My feet also ache and swell."

I deferred prescribing till September 9, when the same was again given, and on September 18 he writes :—" I am pleased to say the sleeplessness at night time has gradually gone away, and I can now sleep much better. I still feel pain in my left leg and foot, but not nearly so bad. I find slight pains at the bottom of my stomach, and also a little more swelling. I still feel weak and unable to walk far at a time, but of course the weather has been very trying even to strong people.

"I am pleased and thankful for the progress I have made, and have to thank you for the splendid results of your treatment. I could not possibly have lived much longer in the terrible suffering I was in."

On September 30 I saw him, and he informed me that after the dose the feet and ankles began to swell, but gradually got better, and that a week ago the right leg felt as if it were bruised, and is now painful and angry-looking—it is swollen and tense, and pits on pressure. He feels, too, when eating, as if the food chokes in the stomach; some flatus, bowels regular.

On this occasion I gave him another dose of the ornith. umbel. The effect of it, however, was to confirm my belief that this swelling of the absorbents, shown by the condition of the right leg and the previous swollen condition of the feet and ankles, resulted from the high pressure put upon the emunctories owing to the setting free of poison in the system.

Subsequently, in a few days, he came in to me in a great fright, and pulling up his trousers showed me the terrible condition, as he thought, of his legs. They were swollen, and great red streaks and patches could be seen coursing down the limbs.

Believing that this was due to the rapid elimination of the cancer poison, I rather astonished him by insisting upon his walking away without any medicine whatever.

Since then, his recovery has gone on uninterruptedly, and though since this last report he has taken two or three doses of the ornithog. umb., he has not had any other medicine (if I except a unit dose of Alliaria officinalis), and is now in the state of health set forth in this letter received from him :—

" Elm Lodge, Feltham, Middlesex.

" May 3, 1899.

" Dr. Cooper.

"DEAR SIR,—In addition to my previous letters to you, I must tell you I have had no pain since the first week in August last; I certainly feel a slight weakness in the stomach at times, but not always.

"My appetite is wonderfully good, and I can eat almost any kind of food, and am also able to enjoy my meals, which I had not done for many years; am able to get about well, and carry on my business without fatigue.

"I have rejoined the Volunteer force and have done two or three good stiff marches, besides firing in competitions, and feel no ill effects. I have never felt so well for nearly twenty years. I feel wonderfully well now, and have gained the two stone odd which I lost during my illness. Everyone I meet, whether in Kensington, Shepherd's Bush, or Feltham, is astonished when they see me, and all speak of the marvellous cure effected by yourself.

"I am, dear Sir,

"Yours faithfully,

"GEO. A. MURRELL."

Evidence could not be stronger in favour of my assertion that these internal cancers are most amenable to treatment; of all the forms of chronic complaints there is no other that so surely deprives the patient of life and in which life can be with such certainty restored by the influence of simple remedies.

This is the lesson of Murrell's case, and his very existence on earth is an undeniable testimony to its import.

In November, 1899, he was examined by a doctor in Brentford for Life Insurance, and notwithstanding the fact of his having been operated upon so recently in the Cancer Hospital, this doctor pronounced him to be absolutely free from diagnosable disease, and recommended him for acceptance at ordinary rates of premium ; that is, in about fifteen months after I had taken him up in a dying state, he is declared by an opinion in no way friendly, to be healthy.

---

[1] Since writing above—June 1900—Murrell has had some return of pain ; this in no way alters argument of text.

CHAPTER III.

Case of Cancer of Liver.—Case of Supposed Cirrhosis of Liver, declared incurable.

THE next are two somewhat similar cases and to these I devote the first portion of this chapter as affording equally important evidence of the truth of my statements.

Both of the patients had been attended by a number of doctors in Southampton.

The first is that of an artist of good repute, whose name, as well as those of the practitioners connected with his case, I suppress for obvious reasons.

On October 29, 1898, I received a letter from this gentleman's wife, from which the subjoined are extracts :—

" Perhaps you will remember whilst in Southampton attending me and bringing me as I thought at the time from the brink of the grave. I wish now to put Mr. M.'s case before you, as no doctor here nor the specialist in London, Dr. M. B., has done any good. At the end of May Mr. M. had jaundice, but got fairly well again in two months, able to walk eight miles. Then as the weather changed he took cold and has been very ill over two months, not able to take any solid food without suffering agonies of pain after it, and is now starving from want, getting thinner and weaker every day.

" Dr. M. B., the specialist, thought there might be a gall stone ; the doctors here a growth or tumour."

The letter went on to ask if I thought it possible to do him any good.

Few particulars as to symptoms having been given, I relied more upon past experience in sending him down Ornith. Umbel. φ A., which he took October 30. On November 2, his wife reported unfavourably ; he had had one of his bad attacks of acidity which had left him more prostrate than any of the preceding ones ; no appetite whatever, takes only a little arrowroot. "To-day he has not been able to touch anything until 4 o'clock p.m., when he took part of an egg beaten up, but without appetite. "I am really afraid," she goes on to say, "he is sinking; he has got very thin and looks dreadfully ill."

The letter went on to request my coming to see him, which I did a few days afterwards, but in the meantime sent down the better indicated remedy, Iris versicolor φ A., and on November 4 report came in "Mr. M. took the powder at 9 this morning, and found it working till 3 o'clock this afternoon, when he was sick naturally, an unusual thing for him; the vomit was slightly acid and yellow, about a teacupful. He is feeling very weak this evening, having been in bed four days and taking no nourishment through the stomach, and he does not feel inclined to take it, being only supported by suppositories."

The assurance of the patient that he felt the remedy to be acting, followed by a change of symptom, in this case a natural sickness, is proof that the selection was the right one.

After this, improvement continued ; the dose was repeated in a week and proved too violent in its action to be pleasant for the patient's comfort ; when disturbance from it ceased, as it did in some hours, improvement again set in for a few days.

The subsequent progress of the case was somewhat checked by a severe cold with feverishness, and on November 27, I again called to see him and was much struck by his jaundiced appearance. This jaundice I ascertained had never really left him since he was seized with it in May. I found the stomach distended, with clearness of percussion over the duodenum except where the left globe of the liver appeared to overlap it, which led me to suspect a carcinomatous growth coming from the under surface of the liver. The patient expressed himself as having been so far wonderfully relieved ; he had been, he said, in agonies of pain for two weeks before adopting my treatment, and had almost wholly lived during this time on food suppositories.

The presence of jaundice and the exacerbation of the symptoms on dark, misty days, led me to select Calend. off. φ A. for him, and after this steady, uninterrupted improvement went on.

Thus, on December 2, his son writes :—"I think since Mr. M. has taken the powder the jaundice is much better ; anyway his colour is much better. There is nothing unusual, as far as we can see, except that the bowels have acted twice a day for the last three days, but have not acted to-day, and his appetite has improved a great deal. This improvement is still maintained, and he has practically left off (food) suppositories."

On December 4, I repeated the Calendula without any disturbance whatever, and towards the close of December I gave him continuous doses of Ferrum picricum 6th dec. in tablets, and subsequently in drops, and without in any way disturbing the continued improvement.

From this absence of disturbance I conclude the greater part of the disease had by this time disappeared.

On February 5, of 1899, the patient himself writes :—
" I am still progressing, having been out and walking about
two or three miles, my legs aching a little, but otherwise
doing well," and his letter goes on : " Now, Sir, I again
thank you for your marvellous treatment. Friends seeing
me down town think it is my ghost, or else I could not
have been so bad as was reported. But I find," he goes
on, " there is a great prejudice against your system and
I wish to testify all I can to its great efficacy."

I care little what nomenclature may be chosen for this
man's disease ; his abdomen had not been opened into
like that of Murrell in the Cancer Hospital, and hence no
one can be absolutely certain whether cancer was present
or not. But one thing is perfectly certain, and this is
that ordinary treatment had altogether failed to afford
relief, and that at the present time the patient is in every
respect in the enjoyment of good health. Beyond a unit
dose of Senecio Doronicum in February, he has not had a
particle of medicine since the above report was made, and
is now quite well.

The next Southampton case is equally interesting; I was telegraphed for on February 10, 1899, to see W. H. M., aged 59, a gentleman connected with the Commissariat Department of the Royal Navy, and supposed to be dying of cirrhosis of the liver. I saw him in the evening of February 10 in the presence of, though not in consultation with, his medical attendant; one of the oldest and most experienced practitioners in the town. I then learned these particulars: twenty-three years ago W. H. M. had had ague in Bombay, had got well, but in 1877 went to Malta when it returned, and has had indefinite symptoms of it ever since. Two years ago was operated on for piles, which he had had since 1882. There is no history of any irregular habits. Present attack began a month ago by his bringing up black blood from his stomach, followed by great pain during the night and next morning, and since then has had occasional sickness, the last time two weeks ago. He has a burning pain all over the chest, under the ribs, and especially round the navel, but present as well throughout the abdomen, with excessive nausea and disinclination for food. Is being entirely fed by the bowel, sleep restless and suffers from pressure across the forehead.   Urine natural.

On examination I found the liver decidedly small, with dulness and hardness in front of the left lobe, but without much distension of the stomach.   I left as medicine a drop or two of an acetous tincture of Lobelia Inflata in a tumbler of water, with orders to take a dessertspoonful every third hour.

This evidently disturbed him, and the report came in next day of general upset and constant pain in hepatic region, and in the left side as well, with increased nausea and sickness ; a suffocating feeling and tightness in the chest; to all of which I replied that he must go on to the unit dose, and that he was not to expect benefit from it for some days. The selection made was Crocus Sativus, which was taken February 12, and soon after the sickness left, but on 18th he complained of pain all over the body under the arm pits, in shoulder blades, up the spine and across the abdomen, with burning on right side, worse round the navel and upwards; from all of which I inferred that the disease was giving out, and consequently I left him without medicine. On the 20th there came in a very good report—food was keeping down and the pain was gone. In this way he went on making good progress, so much so that on March 3 he thus wrote : "My first letter must be to you to tell you that under God's good providence your skilful treatment of my case, so far, has been attended with great success. You will, I know, be as pleased to hear, as I am to tell you, that I am progressing most favourably, have an excellent appetite and enjoy my food, leaving off invariably with an appetite."

Finding such remarkable progress to have been made, I considered there could be no harm, as in the last case, in giving a tablet of Ferrum picricum, 6th dec., every fourth hour, but with the precaution that if he found it upsetting him in any way he was to discontinue it immediately.

5

This I did as the rapid change that had taken place in his symptoms convinced me we were dealing with something very different from ordinary cirrhosis of the liver, and that the growth from the left lobe of the liver was accompanied by a non-cirrhotic shrinkage of the hepatic substance.

The warning was justified by events, for though he did not begin taking the tablets till 8 p.m., at 7 a.m. of the next day copious diarrhœa set in and great prostration, due, as I considered, to the too free elimination of morbid material. Naturally the Ferr. pic. tablets were stopped and medicine again discontinued.

Improvement at once set in, and on March 7 patient wrote : " I am feeling much better, and everyone tells me they see a great improvement within the last week." The letter went on to say that appetite and sleep were good, flatulent pains had left, food was digesting, and except that his legs were weak and his feet and ankles and toes were swollen, he felt very comfortable. This last symptom

I pointed out to him was evidence that the emunctories of the system were at work and the absorbents thrown into increased activity. This proved to be the case, and these swellings soon went down and without the development of any kidney complication.

On March 25 reports : Getting on very well. Swelling of the feet going down, but toes are swollen. Has some scalding pains spreading up from the knees in the muscles with sensitiveness to the touch, and yet a feeling of deadness in them. Bowels were disturbed (from a chill ?) yesterday, stools light-coloured and liquid, and sometimes only flatulent expulsions. Crocus sativus ϕ A. was now given, and on March 28 his daughter wrote :—

"My father is too unwell to write to you. On Sunday he got your letter and dose and took the latter at 1 o'clock p.m. Bowels were disturbed 9.30 p.m. same day, and next day at 1.30 and 8.30 a.m., and several times during the day and again this morning.

"All day yesterday he was feeling most miserable ;

achy, oppressive and drowsy, so much so that he was unable to take anything after his tea at 5 p.m. All through the night he has been in much pain, passing wind, and woke up during the night feeling very sick, with sudden rush of salt water in his mouth; the sickness he managed to stave off, but early this morning it again came on, and he threw up about three pints of very sour and acid stuff. Has had heartburn yesterday and all night, and now severe acid eructations."

The writer goes on :—

"He cannot help thinking the medicines you give him are somewhat too strong for a weak stomach and frame such as his, but of course you know best; he merely wanted to let you know his stomach has always been very weak, and he has never been robust. You will probably get this letter early this afternoon, and if necessary telegraph instructions."

In reply to this I sent a dose of Camphor bromide, 3ru dec., and on April 10 had up a report that for the last day or two he had been much troubled with flatulence and a feeling of soreness and of tightness across the abdomen and the waist, with a full feeling in the chest, and a hot burning sensation in the passages; the swelling of the feet and legs had disappeared for twelve days. Also, the report went on to say that after the Camphor bromide he had had a good night, but much pain and indigestion up to the 3rd and 4th of April (about which time I ordered him a teaspoonful of castor oil every morning), and that since then he had been considerably relieved.

On April 26 patient was able to come up to town by himself to see me, a different man in every respect from what he had been in February; then he was lying prostrate, all medicinal treatment having been discontinued, his state being considered hopeless, and being fed entirely by the bowel; now, though thin, he was sturdy and strong, and able with ease to take this long journey unattended.

As he suffered from a faint, weak feeling before food, and heat and soreness in the pit of the chest, with tendency to looseness of the bowels, I gave a dose of Ornithog. umbel., and he has remained perfectly well ever since. Not a single dose of medicine has he required from that day (April 26, 1899) to this (May, 1900).

It will be evident to the intelligent reader that in dealing with the cancerous affections of the pylorus and adjoining regions we have to do with diseases that are very easily acted on, so easily that the difficulty is to dislodge them in a way commensurate with the patients' safety. Thus in the first of these two cases, that of the artist, I have since been told by him that shortly after I took him in hand—after the dose of Iris versic.—he brought up quite a fair sized pail full of dark glutinous matter, while in that of W. H. M. it is evident that an unmistakable intolerance existed to all but unit doses.

Now when men in an advanced stage of disease go bringing up pails full of thick grumous material it is evident that the process must be very exhausting, and not only so, but that if the channels through which this material has to find an outlet get blocked, a condition obtains that is incompatible with life.

And this is a danger that is present in all advanced types of these diseases; the patients may die though beneficially acted upon. My contention, therefore, is that these diseases can be easily acted upon, and that in our anxiety to bring about recovery, stimulated of course by the same desire on the part of the patient, we must not endeavour to hasten recovery by undue repetition of the remedy.

A very good instance of this is afforded by cancers of the gullet. Here we get an obstruction produced by the narrowing influence of the cancer upon the lumen of the œsophagus. The very moment the remedy acts, as remedies very easily act, upon this affection, a quantity of phlegm, often very offensive, comes away, and the chance for the patient depends upon his allowing this action to expend itself upon the disease. If therefore the physician, blind to Nature's warning, repeats his doses under the old and specious plea "of its being necessary to push the remedy," he will inevitably hasten the death of his patient.   And the more related the dose has been to the disease, the more necessary is it to observe this warning.

What, then, is the upshot of the whole matter?   It is this, that in the diseases of which I have just given examples, the struggle at elimination of the diseased products has almost as much to do with the obstinacy of human nature as with the intractability of the disease to be treated.

Facts are facts, and progress in medicine depends upon putting a right estimate upon these facts, and deducing from them legitimate inferences.

I claim for these facts and the attendant inferences an importance and a power that is provable by the existence in this life of these three men, in the enjoyment of perfect health, who had been declared by leading authorities to be, each one of them, in a dying condition: I refer now to Mr. Murrell, the Southampton artist, and to W. H. M.

CHAPTER IV.

Cancer of the womb: its prevalence.—Depressed spirits inimical to treatment.—Passiveness of mind, not faith, required.—Case of uterine cancer given, greatly relieved. — Another case where operation had failed.—Uterine tumour pressing on rectum where operation was refused, rapid improvement. — Laurocerasus, remarks upon.—Fibrous tumour of the womb: case given.

OF all the diseases that afflict mankind there is none the ravages of which inflict more suffering and distress than this awful present-day scourge. The Sweating Sickness of the middle ages, followed as it was by plague, small-pox and by cholera—all had an immediately terrorising and paralysing effect. But it is doubtful if any one of these very fatal epidemics has in its fell swoop disseminated a tithe of the distress that uterine cancer is insidiously and progressively causing at the present time.

This, however, is not a favourable opportunity for pausing to contemplate the magnitude of this terrible scourge. But it is a very desirable occasion for impressing upon woman-kind the necessity for struggling in every way against indulgence, for it is often nothing but an indulgence, in depression of spirits. We are all products of our Mother Earth, and where, may I ask, on the surface of the globe do we find any living thing—animal or vegetable—when placed in a position suitable to its requirements, living in a way that does not betoken a happy joyousness? The little flower that lifts its face to heaven, no less than the fierce tigress with its cubs, returns thanks to its Creator in manifestation of an innocent contentment.

Should like enjoyment not be forthcoming amongst human beings, it behoves them to carefully study and endeavour to correct an environment that must be inimical to their best interests. The man or woman who succeeds in doing this must necessarily be happy.

The effect of mental depression is more noticeable in the cancers of the womb than in any other form of this shocking scourge. Naturally, too, the action of remedies upon the disease is much more unsatisfactory when sorrow lurks within, and clogs, as it assuredly will, the channels for nutritive material throughout the system. Let it therefore be understood, if I express a favourable opinion upon the power of remedies upon these diseases, that I am free to confess that the greatest successes are gained where the sufferers struggled successfully against mental depression caused by domestic and other worries. The proverbial idea is that a patient must have *faith*; in a sense it is quite true, but equally certain is it that the physician ought to prescribe a remedy such as will give this desirable faith to the patient. For in Medicine faith rests, or ought to rest, upon the evidence of things seen and felt; and it behoves the prescriber to regulate his prescriptions so that as much as possible of this kind of faith may be secured.

The physician who requires his patients to have faith in him before he furnishes them with evidence upon which to found their faith is, to put it mildly, unreasonable. For myself, I admit readily that I seek to cultivate faith in my patients, and the instrument, and the only instrument I employ, is what appeals rationally and soberly to their senses—a vital force working upon a vital force. My reason for introducing these considerations at the present juncture is to give me the opportunity of frankly acknowledging that my advice to all patients suffering from chronic disease is to remain perfectly passive in mind when first coming under treatment.

A treatment that begins by endeavouring to secure a patient's confidence is a humbugging affair ; but a treatment that ends by the establishment of a patient's faith by relief of his sufferings is one that aims at a natural sequence of events. The best thing a doctor can do to a patient who enters his study in a querulous and suspecting frame of mind, both for his own and his patient's benefit, is to show them the hall-door, or, as the French would say, *donner la clef des champs*. A seriousness and determination to get cured is almost as necessary as an equally serious determination on the doctor's part to effect a cure.

In the complaints of women, but particularly in uterine cancers, the need for complete passiveness of mind in the commencement of treatment must be insisted upon.

Cancer complaints of all varieties and in every situation seem to feed upon depressing emotions. Equally true is it that half our sorrows are self-inflicted, and therefore ought to be carefully guarded against.

In the first edition of this work I brought forward a case of undoubted cancer of the womb; it was one in which the husband introduced the case to me in this letter :—

" 24-2-99.

" DEAR SIR,—Having heard through Mr. M. of your treatment of his disease, I venture to write concerning my wife, who is suffering from cancer of the womb. Three years ago we thought she was suffering from change of life. She was examined by Dr. B. of this town, and he told her there was nothing the matter, only change of life, but that the left lip of the womb was swollen. It has been going on like this ever since until last November, when she was examined by Dr. J. and Dr. T., and they both pronounced it cancer. They advised her to go to Brompton Road Hospital. She was there fourteen days, and was examined by Dr. B. J. under ether; he told her he could do nothing and sent her home, and told her to live as quietly as possible. . . . .

" I was overjoyed when I heard from Mr. M. about you; I thought there was one more chance for my poor dear wife. I must tell you her appetite is fairly good. Her spirits were always good, but lately she gets very low, and I often come home from work and find that she has been or is crying. . . . ."

And in a postscript to his letter he writes :—" Dr. J. said

he could not operate because the cancer had attached itself to the bladder, and to cut it away would be almost certain death."

On February 27, 1899, I sent Helleb. Vir. φ A, with a request for monthly reports. On March 23 came a report that "the ninth day after the dose, a bright red discharge set in, mixed with very dark, stringy, clotted blood ; at the same time I [the patient] had severe pains in my hips and back, and a sort of bearing down ; could not stand or walk and was obliged to go to bed ; it lasted for a few days, and I was then able to come down again. And so it has worked at five different times during the month, and between each interval I felt a little better within myself. But I still at times feel a kind of stinging, but not nearly so sharp as it was before taking the powder ; the stinging seems to work more towards my back passage ; yesterday I felt a slight pain going towards my left breast. So, sir, [she goes on] you see I have improved ; now, do you think you would like to see me ? "

On April 10 the patient came up to see me, and expressed herself in the most joyful terms owing to her greatly improved feelings. A good deal of bloody and white discharge had come on during the previous week, and a feeling as if something were working about in the rectum and bowels; " is still restless at night, but the pains are less severe."

Local examination was certainly not so assuring as the patient's testimony; the parts were bathed in blood, which seemed to come principally from two large granular masses that hung down on either side of the *os uteri* from a hard and fixed fundus. Further examination than this was undesirable, owing to the free hæmorrhage. Three days after seeing her I sent Caltha palustris ϕ A, and since then have had most favourable reports; in that of April 30 the patient writes :—" On fourth day after the powder, pains set in in my hips, especially the left hip; and on fifth day red but not *bright* red discharge as before, a yellow-red discharge, and not smooth and stringy but gritty, no clots, and it lasted only one day.

" The white discharge continues ; I think the bladder has slightly improved, the probing, shooting pain is less ; have felt some of it in left breast this last two weeks, very little of it towards rectum."

The breaking-down remedy in this instance was undoubtedly the Green Hellebore. Helleborus Niger Fœtidus, and Viridis, are remarkable for the production of an overpowering depression, accompanied by the fearful sense of sinking at the pit of the chest and all over the body, with laxity and enfeeblement of the muscular system and a sense of blank despair such as we meet with in the cancers, especially in scirrhous cancers. The Helleb. Viridis I find to be more pronounced in its effects on internal cancers than the Helleb. Nig., and both are certainly very often called for in cancer cases.

The Helleb. Nig. shows its full power in certain forms of facial lupus, and in old and obstinate ulcerations of the legs.

This patient has, I am given to understand, undergone

a great deal of distress and serious domestic worry since this report was written, but she still, up to the time of writing, is able to keep about, and enjoy a great measure of activity. Treating a case like this at a distance, and under the most unfavourable circumstances possible, is not conducive to recovery. This patient cannot in all probability get well, poor thing, but most certainly her life has been prolonged by treatment, and with few exceptions, she has been able to do without morphia.

While I write (May, 1900), there comes to hand a most unexpectedly gratifying account, to the effect that on the thirteenth day after the last powder (Helleb. fæt.) a clot, of which an admirable drawing was sent, and which represented the moulding of the cavity of the womb, came away, the patient describing it as "a most curious clot ; it was in some parts over an inch thick, and it was lined with white veins, and measured about six inches."

Evidently great relief has followed, as she writes only of *slight* pricking and shooting. This certainly is satisfactory.

The relief given to this patient was so great that a lady aged 62, living close at hand, and who suffered from a similar malady, came up to consult me. Briefly her case ran: Six years ago had a complication of ailments, diarrhœa, asthma, &c., and had to lie up five or six months. Then a fibroid tumour of the womb was diagnosed, but a year after, though suffering from hæmorrhage, the tumour could not be felt. A year ago she passed long fungoid-looking masses and clots of blood, and was declared to have cancer of the womb, and to be incurable. Operation was tried by one of the first operators in London, and proved unsuccessful, and it was found impossible to remove all the growth. At the time of consulting me on May 6, 1899, she was having antikamnia tablets, as the injections of morphia had disagreed so frightfully with her. Her symptoms were great back-ache, and bearing down from a feeling of weight, chiefly on the right side, and much pain round the navel, with sinking in the pit of the chest, slight constipation, but no dysuria.

This patient has, of course, required a good deal of treatment; this has not been essentially different from that adopted in other cases, Crocus Satinus and Vernalis, Helleborus Niger, Laurocerasus, and other remedies have been given as the symptoms indicated, and now I am pleased to say the lady is in the enjoyment of really good health; digestion and strength are good, and there has been no loss of flesh. With one exception, last September, when she had a good deal of suffering for a week, she has been almost free from pain. Surely a treatment like this is better than operation or morphia drugging. It is not to be supposed that cases which have gone so far as this had can be cured.

If, in the last case, there is little to be learned, in the next there is, on the contrary, a very great deal of valuable instruction.

A. C., aged 54, married 30 years, nullipara, miscarriage 10 years after marriage, subject up to two years ago to bilious attacks from the age of 17, has been under treatment for four years for uterine hæmorrhage, but not till two years ago was a growth from the wall of the uterus detected.   Operation was discountenanced, the tumour being evidently thought malignant, and this by a foremost consultant in women's diseases.   The consulting surgeon, of, I believe, the Samaritan Hospital, was then consulted, but declined operation on consultation with others.   The symptoms are simply hæmorrhage, going on every day, generally bright in colour, has only a few hours' interval in the twenty-four, and last week was practically excessive.   Much back-ache, and pain with the clots, and feels the tumour pressing upon the bowel.   Much constipation, for which she has to take medicine, and restless sleep from the back-ache.   Lately pain in left shoulder and behind left breast.   On local examination a very weighty mass was found pressing down into the passage.   That the case was considered one of great urgency is evident from the fact that her medical attendant declared that colotomy would soon have to be performed.

On January 5, 1900, I prescribed Laurocerasus φ A, and a pill every night of 3 grs. of simple ox gall.

On January 19, came the very cheery intelligence that though she had had much pain night and day for the first week, for the second had less pain than for two years; and that, whereas formerly she felt ill and uncomfortable when the pain lessened, this was not now at all the case. Still has back-ache, but pains in the left shoulder and breast are gone—*Nil*.

On February 2, reports:—From January 22 to 26 had much pain, and on the night of 23rd much acid vomit came up, with fainting feeling across abdomen and left side up to the head; hæmorrhage for two or three days, but no clots as she used to have in quantities. Is much stronger, though bowels are more confined. The dose of January 5 again.

February 16.—Has been much better up to 13th, and then passed clots, but much less than before treatment; these are sometimes dark, but sometimes bright, and are accompanied by back-ache; the act of walking causes pain over left thigh and groin, but still can walk much better, and it does not bring on hæmorrhage. Crocus Sativ. φ A was then given, and her report thereupon is very significant. On the same evening had a great deal of pain across the lower back, and slept but little that night and the next, and on third night had cramp in the stomach as well as back-ache and diarrhœa, and since this has been much better. No medicine was given on this occasion, and when seen a month afterwards she declared herself better than she had been for four years. It is unnecessary to follow the treatment further. When seen on May 4 she was feeling in every way improved, was walking about in perfect comfort, and except that she still felt weak with dyspnœa on going up heights, and that there was still some oozing discharge, she was without the slightest suffering.

I have stated that this case was instructive; it is a very good example of how easy it is to discard the truly curative remedy. Instead of relieving the pain, the Laurocerasus caused her to have much more suffering for the first week, and had I proposed to see her in three or four days instead of in a fortnight, the chances are the right remedy would probably have been discontinued and another selected in its stead. This is why one practitioner gets good results where another, more anxious and more apprehensive, fails, even though he may use the same remedy.

This is a favourable opportunity for giving the leading indications for Laurocerasus. A sense of fatigue pervades the whole system, with a very painful condition of the hard and indurated tissue of the parts affected, this pain being in general much ameliorated by sleep; there is a tendency to an oozing of blood that is most generally bright and mixed with gelatinous clots. This applies to chest as well as to uterine and rectal symptoms, only that the blood comes painlessly into the mouth but with great pain *per vaginam*.

In most cases it will be found that the pains it relieves are ones that start from the lower part of the spine and extend either round the pelvis or up to the head, and are accompanied by a sense of suffocation, and a sick feeling, with drowsiness, and a great desire for sleep that *generally* brings relief; in cases that are sleepless the desire for sleep is very great. The digestion is weak, the bowels are confined, the patient is low-spirited, with flatulence and burning in the chest after food, and a constant tired, sick feeling, the entire frame being enfeebled, and inclined to loss of flesh and hæmorrhages that are small in quantity and bright in colour. Its flatus is audible and gurgling, and rolls about the upper abdomen.

These instances of benefit from treatment are quite sufficient to establish a claim for arborivital remedies, when prescribed according to the symptoms, as being remedial in the severest possible cases, even in the most painful cancers.

That the fibrous tumours of the womb should also fall

under their sway is natural to expect. These tumours are less malignant in their tendency than the true cancers. As old age advances, they often develop malignant characters, according to Dr. Herbert Snow,[1] who thus writes:—" The same holds good (*i.e.*, tendency to malignancy) to a more limited extent with uterine myomata, the familiar fibroids. Some eventually pass into sarcomata. And though many assuredly do not, even in extreme old age, it is yet likely that with more careful observation at women's hospitals (where pathology as a rule is not a strong point), the sequence will prove far less rare than is now held."

The statement that pathology, as a rule, is not a strong point at women's hospitals is very amusing. I expect next to learn that theology is not a strong point among Bishops !

That some of the worst of these cases do not become malignant is evident from this case, taken from my work

---

[1] " Cancerous and other Tumours," p. 25.   London : Baillière, 1898.

on "Serious Diseases Saved from Operation," p. 13-17, now out of print.

IMMENSE FIBROID TUMOUR (OF THE WOMB) GIVING RISE TO GREAT PAIN.—Close by where this child (referred to before) lived was a very interesting case, about which the same lady wrote, asking me to recommend an institution in town in which this woman could be operated upon.

As this woman, Mrs. A., was then suffering intense pain, I advised her taking some remedies for the pain before thinking of an operation. Her case, in reply to a letter from me, ran thus :—

" *October* 16, 1895.

" SIR,—Many thanks for your kind letter received this morning. I must say that in the first place I have a fibrous tumour in the womb, which I have had for years and at times suffered very much with.

" In May, 1887, I had a disease fall on my eyes (glaucoma), and was in the Royal Westminster Ophthalmic

Hospital, Chandos Street. There I had one eye operated upon, and had them bad for some time. Then they wanted to take the eye out, but I felt I could not have that done. I was then advised to go to the London Homœopathic Hospital, which I did in June, and very thankful I am that I did, for after a time they got much better.

"About two years after, as an in-patient at the same hospital with the other eye, I got better without any operation.

"Now as regards this last trouble. It was six weeks ago last Friday—I had previously been feeling very unwell, not an unusual thing with me—I was taken with intense pain in the pit of the stomach, seemed like being drawn up with cords, then shooting pains through my breasts and up under my arms, and through to my back, that lasted four hours; after that I was easy for about an hour or two, then they came on again about half-past eight and lasted till three o'clock; then I was sick and brought up a great deal that smelt very bad indeed; then I was two or three days and had another attack, then stopped a week; then another, and so on until last Sunday. Then I had one in the afternoon, and another in the evening, and another on Monday afternoon, and yesterday, one in the afternoon and another in the evening; but yesterday I could not bring anything up to speak of. After the vomiting I get ease at once and am quite exhausted and can go to sleep directly. Then another thing is, I have had the most dreadful irritation all over my body, but more especially in the palms of my hands and the soles of my feet, and at times it seems quite unbearable; not anything to be seen, but the skin is very dry and hot.

" Another thing is the urine, which is very deep colour and very yellow."

The letter goes on to express her conviction of its being necessary to go into hospital, and concludes by saying :—

" I had a very restless and sleepless night last night, and am feeling sick this morning; very little appetite and almost afraid to take anything."

However, instead of going into a hospital, all these pains so far lessened under treatment that on December 3, 1895, she was able to come up and see me, and then I found that she was suffering from an immense tumour, that by its weight alone was dragging her down fearfully, and which filled the entire upper pelvis and lower abdomen.

Her age was 58, and the change of life had taken place twelve years back, at which time she had begun to suffer; and it was then that the tumour was discovered, and was supposed to have existed much longer. Her present state is as follows :—

Continual pain and weight in the pit of the chest, less in the morning ; gets worse after taking food, has to loosen her clothes and lie down. The attacks of pain were more severe before taking my remedies, but now they hang about more ; she has less sickness and consequently less relief from her distress. Scarcely ever gets a night's rest ; dreadful irritation all over the body—hands and all—worse at night. Warmth brings it on. Bowels acting.

The real treatment of the case may be said to have now begun. I explained to her the serious nature of her disease, and how very simple my treatment would be, did she elect to remain under me; that the only alternative was a serious operation, for which, as she was now in town, she could make arrangements, and that for myself I naturally advised a pursuance of the same treatment as had already been partly adopted, although her case would put medicinal treatment to the severest possible test. She elected to remain under me, and I began by giving Atropa Belladonna φ A, with a prescription for Magnesia Carbonica CC. Two tablets every third hour if in pain.

December 20, 1895.—Is very much better; for three days has not had sufficient pain to necessitate taking the tablets. Has been much on her feet lately, which has caused great bearing down. *Nil.*

January 27, 1896.—Up to two weeks ago was better, but since then has had pain every day, and the tablets do not relieve as they did. Last Saturday had a very bad turn after dinner (early), which lasted till nine o'clock, and was very sick, and now irritation is as bad as ever. Last night never slept the whole night through.

Sent Daphne Mezereum ɸ A.

After this the irritation of the skin improved, but the pain returned and she was much troubled with flatus, for which treatment was given with more or less relief. On April 20 she still complained of great pain with retching, and sickness, and irritation of the skin, all the symptoms being worse after meals.

For this Cephaelis Ipec. ɸ A, was given, and it is no exaggeration to say that since then she has made an almost uninterrupted and a truly marvellous recovery.

I have heard but twice directly from her since April, but indirectly get constant reports. One of these times that she herself wrote was on May 25, 1896, and her letter runs thus :—

"I heard from Mrs. D. the other day, and she told me

that you thought I ought to write oftener to you; why I do not is because I am careful not to trouble you more than I can possibly help and until I feel much worse. I feel better and am quite sure your treatment is doing me good; I am less in size and have the pain less, can eat better and not feel so sick. Is not all this very encouraging?"

The next occasion of her writing to me was on June 17, 1896, when she asked for medicine as she had had some threatenings of pain.

A mutual friend writes under date January 23, 1897:—

"I saw Mrs. A., who is better than she has been for years; has had hardly any pain for a month or more; she says it is wonderful, she is almost afraid of speaking of it."

Here, then, is a case literally snatched from the knife of the surgeon; the patient is very thankful, but there the matter ends.

The patient above referred to has been seen by me, but

once since, when she came, about a year ago, with a feeling of great bearing down in the pelvis. This was obviously due to the contracted tumour finding its way into the pelvic cavity. On this account I advised her to let matters drift, especially as her health was otherwise excellent, and a few weeks ago I received intelligence of her being in perfect health.

Mrs. A. lives, or lived until lately, at Horsham, and can verify every word of the above report.

Our hospitals could not exist if such patients were treated at home in this simple way, consequently such treatment does violence to existing interests.

CHAPTER V.

Anæmic ulceration of the Stomach.—Malignant ulceration; two cases.—Gastric ulceration threatening malignancy.—Ornithogalum Umbellatum; short remarks upon.

THIS chapter is chiefly made up from a paper that appeared in *The Homœopathic World*, April 1898; it is here reprinted with some few additions.

ARBORIVITAL MEDICINE.

It would be impossible to adduce more striking and more satisfactory evidence of the great power possessed by plant remedies, irrespective of any special mode of preparation, than is afforded by the following cases:—

CASE I.—ULCERATION (ANÆMIC) OF THE STOMACH.

The first case is that of a Sister of Mercy, aged 30, date of coming, November 15, 1897, in whom a strong anæmic history existed, and with whom sickness of stomach had prevailed for some twelve years. The symptoms began at eighteen years of age with anæmia and cessation of menstruation for six months; since then the monthly period ceased on one occasion for about the same time, and now nothing has been seen for $2\frac{1}{2}$ years. She used to have a good deal of left submammary pains, but this is now only felt occasionally. Her principal symptom is that after meals a weight is felt in the stomach; this goes on till froth comes in her mouth with much clear fluid, and then her food is vomited, bringing with it great relief. Stomach sometimes very distended, generally in the morning, and lately the feeling after food has been more of an emptiness than of a weight. Feels frightfully depressed when these sensations come on. Bowels are regular, but for two years suffered from obstinate constipation; there is no melæna, and no uterine bearing down, or leucorrhœa.

Actæa racemosa φ *A, given.*—A friend brings the report to me (November 29) that the sister " has been much better till last night, when she felt swollen and was unable to eat anything this morning."

Reported also having been sick on Saturday the 27th, after dinner, the only time within the fortnight. Her spirits are much better, and the principal thing she now complains of is being very flatulent with a sour taste as from fermentation and as if everything turned acid.

For this last symptom I did not think it necessary to alter the selection, and gave again Actæa rac. φ A.

One of her fellow sisters reports (February 15, 1898) that in every way improvement has gone on, and that to all appearances she is in perfect health, though the catamenia are still absent.

In selecting the remedy I had more in view the past symptoms than the present state of the patient. The submammary pain had formerly been a prominent symptom, and this, with anæmia and tendency to irregularity of the menstrual functions, was characteristically an Actæa condition.

She has remained perfectly well.

CASE II.—ULCERATION OF STOMACH, APPARENTLY MALIGNANT.

Miss J., aged 50, a thin, spare, drawn-featured woman. Date of case, November 6, 1897. Fifteen years ago vomited blood, and dates her sufferings from this, but has always been subject to gastric pain.

Symptoms : Pains in the stomach, with sickness ; vomiting two or three times a day ; feels a pressure in every nerve of the body, sometimes in one part, sometimes in another, with pain across the chest, sometimes after food, sometimes at night, and sometimes on an empty stomach ; a great deal of wind and sometimes a swollen feeling across the lower chest; occasional heartburn with rising of food ; nasty canker taste in the morning ; sleep not good from the pains; wandering dreams; bowels are confined. Previous treatment has been at the Kilburn Dispensary, under several doctors, at a homœopathic dispensary, and at a principal homœopathic hospital. Ornithogalum Umbellatum ♦ A. was prescribed.

November 13.—Not sick since Monday the 8th, but still has pains; the pressure pains are bad; the pain in the lower chest is constant, but it is better at night than before dose; wakes in perspirations at night — a new feature; still dreams; pressure across lower chest same; heartburn and nasty taste much better; bowels confined. *Nil.*

November 27.—Has been much better, but to-day had a good deal of pain across the chest when coming here; worse on left side; perspirations at night are less; "goes cold before the pains;" no heartburn, but nasty taste still and confined bowels. Again Ornith. Umb. ⚥ A.

December 11.—Pain across chest much better; perspirations less; coldness same; had much looseness of the bowels next day, after dose; they continued acting three or four times a day for a week; sleeps better and dreams less. *Nil.*

January 19, 1898. Very much better in every way; food keeps down well; vomiting about twice a week; perspiration less; bowels confined. *Nil.*

February 8.—Looks a different woman; has not been once sick; still has some discomfort, but able to bear the pains better; mouth and throat are dry in the morning. Unit dose repeated of Ornith. Umb.

The Ornithogalum Umb. is a species of garlic (*Allium Sativum*), and, like it and Allium Cepa, produces indigestion with excessive eructations of wind.   (See p. 87.)

The sister of this patient has, since this report was written, died of cancer of the stomach.   I had not treated her.

This patient has on about three occasions, since the above report was taken, required a dose of the Ornith. Umb. for pain, and when seen (May, 1899), was in almost perfect health.

CASE III.—ULCERATION OF THE STOMACH, APPARENTLY

MALIGNANT.

My third case is in many respects like the last.   A lady asked me to prescribe for the following :—

Mrs. K., aged 62, living at Hammersmith, a widow, a poor tailoress. Date of case January, 1898. Last summer twelvemonth was seized with profuse vomiting of blood and melæna and became very ill. For a fortnight lay unconscious; her lips only kept moist by ice and brandy, "but was fed artificially." After long months of illness gradually recovered, but has lived since on milk and slops and Quaker Oats.

Is now again threatened with the same symptoms, having lately spat up clots of blood, and feels whenever she turns in bed as if a bag of liquid turns also. Her doctor says it is gastric ulcers and that she will never be cured, but by care may live some time longer. Suffers much with swollen feet and legs and inability to walk with any ease about her work. Her mother, aunt and brother died of cancer. January 12, 1898, gave Ornith. Umb. ⚬ A.

On January 23, 1898, lady writes:—"Mrs. K. sent me word she took the dose on 12th, and that she could hardly believe it possible it was the powder which had made her feel so much better. I [the lady] heard again from her stating that she continued to improve, and last Friday I called to see her and found her looking so bright and so much stronger. She told me that all that oppression at her stomach was gone, and the 'fluid sack,' as she described it, that rolled about in her inside had seemed to go down, and she felt nothing of it now, and the symptom that particularly struck her [the writer] was the cheeriness, the freedom from oppression that made her feel so light."

Nothing more was given, and on February 10 report came in that she was not feeling so well again, has the same symptoms on the right as on the left side of stomach; a great oppression and a drawing sensation just as she used to feel for a long time before the vomiting of blood came. Again Ornith. Umb. ⚹ A.

On February 17 I received this letter :—

"DEAR DR. COOPER,—Mrs. K. walked here to see me

yesterday morning looking really well, with a colour in her cheeks. She told me she had received from you another wonderful powder, which she had taken, and almost immediately afterwards had felt another woman. The drawing pains had ceased, and the dreadful feeling of oppression and illness had been almost immediately relieved. She said she had gone about her work singing, and felt light and happy, and the bag of fluid which she describes as wobbling about in her stomach had gone down into quietness, &c. She really looked so well that I think she must be curable. Do you not think so? The change in her appearance yesterday was so great from the time before when I saw her."

March 11, 1898.—Report received: Mrs. K. is keeping perfectly well.

No further report came to hand till November 2, 1899, when the patient returned, complaining of a drawing sensation in the stomach and a general feeling of gastric discomfort; otherwise her health had been very good.

This went away at once on the exhibition of the above remedy. Considering that she reached her 66th birthday in March of this year (1900) this is eminently satisfactory.

These cases tell their own tale; they need no further comment. I simply give the facts, and readers may put whatever construction they please upon them.

The next case is reported for the first time :—

GASTRIC ULCERATION, THREATENED MALIGNANCY.

Florence F., aged 22, (date of case, May 12, 1898), was treated in the London Hospital when 17 years old for anæmia and sickness of stomach; remained for seven weeks under treatment and then returned to work, only to knock up again, however, for a year after had to go into the London Temperance Hospital with the same symptoms and with gastric hæmorrhage in addition. Gastric ulceration was then diagnosed.

Remained for five or six weeks in hospital and then went to the country; after this resumed work but had to knock off from a seizure of scarlet fever.

Following this, gastric symptoms again began ; was treated at home, but unsuccessfully, and was obliged to seek admission to University College Hospital. This was two years ago.   Here she remained for seven weeks and then was transferred to a Convalescent Home at East-bourne, where she remained on milk diet for a month. Again she resumed work, but was obliged to give up and go into a Home at St. Leonards, and from this again to the University College Hospital, and after a three weeks' stay in hospital again returned to work in the country until the November previous to my seeing her.   Then, for the third time, received admission into the University College Hospital, and remained under treatment till she again went as an in-patient of the Hospital at Eastbourne (Princess Alice's) for ten weeks. Then again came to town where she has been getting worse and worse for the last month.

Symptoms.—Great pain after eating, from the pit of the stomach through to the back, with violent retching;

submammary stitch, worse when she retches. Had haematemesis within the last seven weeks. The pain in the pit of the chest goes on constantly; had to put on mustard leaves to assuage it last night.

Monthly periods irregular, four months since the last.

Comes over faint with a taste of blood in mouth when attempting to eat, has headache across the eyes with a hammering in the head going from the forehead to the occiput and coming on irregularly.

Actæa. Rac. φ A. prescribed. A week after, reports that she has been throwing up everything. Dose repeated.

June 23, 1898.—Much improved the last few weeks; only is much constipated; food keeps down much better.

Ferr. Phos. 3 x. 3 ij., two grains thrice daily.

July 7.—Is much better, can eat meat now which she had not been able to do since seventeen years of age, has been having nose-bleed for two or three days. Monthly periods still irregular and is constipated Spiræa Ulmar. φ A.

July 27.—Keeping down food well, but has occasional nose-bleed and also pain in stomach.   Ferr. Phos. I x., one grain in single dose.

September 15.—Gets sick if attempts work, and bowels are still confined.   Up to this time general improvement had gone on, but it is evident it was not complete; the long continued delicacy had told its tale and had sadly enfeebled the digestive organs.

It was at this juncture, I gave her a unit dose of Ornithogal. Umbel., and shortly afterwards she went into service and has since got on perfectly well.

It may be well to interpose some remarks upon this very interesting plant—

ORNITHOGALUM UMBELLATUM.

"The *Ornith. Umbellat.* (*vide* Treasury of Botany, *Art.* ORNITHOGALUM : London, Longmans) is a common weed in many parts of England and Scotland.   It is known as the Star of Bethlehem from its being abundant in Palestine

and having star-like flowers.   It is also supposed to be the
Dove's Dung of Scripture (2 Kings ch. vi.); and its bulbs,
which are wholesome and nutritious when cooked, are
eaten to this day in Palestine.   The genus is closely allied
to Scilla, from which it is distinguished only by its flowers
being persistent instead of deciduous, and white greenish
or yellowish instead of blue.   All the species are bulbous
plants, with radical and not stem-sheathing leaves, and
terminal racemes of flowers, each flower with a withered
bract beneath it.   Their perianth has six distinct seg-
ments, spread out star-fashion; and their six stamens
have flattened filaments, and are almost free from the
perianth."

Belonging to the natural order Liliaceæ it is botanically
allied to Asparagus Officinalis, Paris Quadrifolia, Convallaria
Majalis, Scilla Maritima, Agraphis Nutans, Colchicum
Autumnale, Allium Sativum, Allium Cepa, and Polygona-
num Officinale, besides of course many other less known
but valuable remedies.

My acquaintance with it in cancer cases was due to the very distinctive disturbance it produced in a woman very sensitive to all alliaceous flavouring substances in food. The dose was taken at midday, and the same evening distension of the stomach and duodenum came on, with frequent belching of mouthfuls of offensive flatus obliging her to loosen her clothes, and this was accompanied by the most hateful depression of spirits and desire for suicide, a feeling of complete prostration and painful sinking across the pit of the chest, and a feeling of sickness that kept her awake the greater part of the night, and that did not pass off for several days.

The subject of this disturbance was about 54 years of age, of quite a sanguine temperament, inclined to enfeebled digestion, and with a history of pleuritic seizures, and a possible phthisical tendency, but otherwise not subject to any settled form of disease, and not sensitive to remedies.

Since the medicinal thrill above recorded her general

strength, digestion and capacity for the enjoyment of life have manifestly improved.

The Ornith. Umb. in those sensitive to it goes at once to the Pylorus, causes painful spasmodic contraction of it, and distends the duodenum with flatus, its pains being invariably increased when the food attempts to pass the pyloric outlet of the stomach. Depression of spirits, a sick and faint feeling before food, with pain, heat and soreness in the pit of the chest, and a suffocating feeling and pain under the arm-pits, in the shoulders and spine, offensive flatus constantly rising and coated tongue and tendency to diarrhœa, with a feeling of want of support in nephritic regions, and a weak feeling in the knees will call for it.

Agonising feeling in the chest and stomach, starting from the pylorus with a flatus that rolls in balls from one side to the other, loss of appetite, phlegmmy retchings, and loss of flesh, also point to it.

CHAPTER VI.

Cancer, internal and external: in contrast.—Case of Cancer in both neck and breast.—Case of Breast-Cancer.—The treatment of abdominal cancer quite different from that of the breast. —Ferrum picricum in Warty Growths.—Two cases of Lupoid Warts.

THE division of cancer into internal and external is not one that will meet with the approval of the modern scientist, who is nothing if not a pathologist.

As no road is worthy of the name that does not lead to Earl's Court, so no classification of disease is worthy of consideration that does not meet the requirements of pathology; nevertheless, this simple classification into internal and external cancers is an absolutely necessary one when the question of the curability of the disease has to be considered.

The cases given show that the breaking down of many

of the internal cancers is a very simple affair indeed, and that satisfactory evidence is readily obtainable of the possibility of effecting this desirable result.

The evidence of the influence of unit doses upon the external forms of cancer, of which the cancers of the breast form by far the larger proportion, is by no means so completely satisfactory; the cancers of external parts, speaking very broadly, require a longer period of time before the tremendous power of the arborivital doses manifests itself by evident diminution in size, and moreover, it is more difficult to get the cancer germs, pent up as they are in the form of swellings, to disperse when thus localised.

This statement is left as written; it requires qualification. It is perfectly accurate as regards breast cancers, but in the scirrhous swellings of the neck, I find as proved by the next case as well as that reported at p. 15, that remedies act very promptly, though even then a curative issue is not always assured.

It is from numerous observations that I draw the conclusion that cancer, especially in a cumulated form, can be easily acted on, and that if the practitioner wishes to disperse it he must exercise great delicacy of manipulation, so to speak, with his remedies. Above all things he must give the disease *rest*, a rest particularly from medicine; which is really another way of saying with Hahnemann, that as long as the action of the remedy continues, it ought not to be interfered with.[1]

Take, for example, this experience. A lady, at the age of 73 years, sought my advice under these circumstances. She had on the left side of the neck a scirrhous cancer, which had existed for some twenty years, and upon which she had had a severe blow six years before. The effect of the blow was to cause this growth—which before had been steadily increasing in size—to diminish, but

---

[1] "Chronic Diseases," by S. Hahnemann, vol. i., p. 155. New York, Radde, 1845.

along with its diminution came a swelling of the same nature in her right breast.

The breast then took an action and began gradually increasing, until it was large and pendulous and heavy, and threatened to burst ; so much so that her medical adviser told her that operation was peremptorily called for, and that her only chance of living depended upon her being operated upon within a week.

It was at this juncture she sought my advice, making use of these words :—" I am now 73 years of age, and naturally have not very much longer to live, but while life lasts I do not wish to be mutilated."

My advice was to place herself under what I believed to be a natural treatment of disease, and that though I could not promise that a large mass of cancer could at her time of life ever be eliminated from the system, I yet could assure her the probabilities were she might live two or three years longer, and perhaps even die of something quite different from cancer. I took care at the same time to warn her that there might often come reasons for misgivings, but that if she made up her mind to try my treatment, I would expect her, come what would, to remain under it to the end.

It is unnecessary to go into details of this lady's case, suffice it to say that shortly after coming under the arborivital remedies the size of the cervical swelling rapidly went down, and that of the breast as rapidly increased.

The warning, therefore, I had given not to be frightened, applied to both doctor and patient thus early in the treatment, but for myself I felt confident that this effect on the cervical swelling must be beneficial, and that if the breast did increase, it could not be from an action other than a favourable one, and that in all probability the breast, though it threatened, would not burst. The subsequent progress entirely confirmed my suspicions, and it is with the greatest possible gratification that I am now enabled to state that this lady has reached her 79th year, in the enjoyment of health and happiness, as far as her sensations go; that the breast cancer, though it certainly has from time to time threatened to burst, has not done so, and is at present diminishing in size; that the swelling of the neck is hardly perceptible, and that the lady has never had a day's illness in bed since she first adopted this treatment, four years ago. As she herself truly remarks, were she now to die of cancer, it would be with a sense of thankfulness that she had not been operated on.

I have it from friends of hers that her former medical attendant continually inquires about her, and expresses himself astonished at her being still alive.

Extracts from this patient's recent letters may be interesting :—

On February 27, 1899, she writes: " I am feeling much better since I took your last powder.

" The swelling has remained perfectly quiet and stationary so far as I (the patient) can judge. My appetite is fairly good, I sleep well, and am as strong as I could expect to be at my advanced age."

And on May 8 she writes :—

" My report to-day, being a very good one, shall be very brief. In every respect I am feeling better, and the swelling has not caused me any uneasiness since I last wrote."

This, then, is the present condition of a patient who, in December next, will be 79 years of age, and who, at the age of 73, was to have been operated on for a scirrhous breast, and whose case had been advised upon by Paget and other well known authorities, without the slightest hope having ever been held out to her, of being able to avoid an operation.

The arborivital doses have not caused a removal of the disease, but they have kept it in abeyance, have almost entirely removed the pain, and have enabled the patient to reach an advanced age with hardly a moment's apprehension of any kind.

Thus ran the report of this very interesting case in the first edition of this book; the sequel will naturally be expected.

In April and May of 1899, she contracted a severe cold with bronchitis, but happily pulled round wonderfully. Though weakened she gradually regained her strength, and towards the close of November she reported to me a very noteworthy incident. About this time she felt "a working" and a pulling in the situation of what had been the cervical swelling; it seemed to her as if the roots of the swelling were being dragged out and were taking their departure. This evidently was the case, for there is no longer a trace of cervical swelling.

But close upon the disappearance of this scirrhous mass came a simultaneous swelling of the right breast. It rapidly increased in size, it moved round the side of the chest to under the arm, it became terribly heavy, turned black on the surface, and threw out great dusky prominences on its pendulous surface.

These blackish swellings soon began discharging a clear but most offensive fluid, from openings from the size of a sixpence to a half-crown. This discharge, apparently the cancer-juice itself, has gone on pouring away copiously from the end of November till now; and as I write the following letter reaches me from a lady friend in daily attendance.

"*May* 14, 1900.

"DEAR SIR,—I am again writing to report Mrs. H.'s condition, which does not seem to alter much from week to week. Her breast is still about the same, fresh places rising and discharging, principally a watery fluid; the discharge is still very copious and unpleasant.

"*The breast looks much smaller* and not quite so appalling to the sight.

"Her general health is good, she sleeps and eats well, though she is now again troubled with constipation."

There is therefore, every appearance, every likelihood, I

had almost said, of this enormous mass of cancer disappearing altogether.

Neither the patient nor I myself expected at one time that she would survive this great draining away; but from the above report, and with other facts of the case before me, I almost expect her to reach her 80th birthday, and should she do so, it will be but with slight remains of her old enemy. Well may one say of her, that she who will endure to the end, the same shall be saved! Life is, I need not say, very uncertain as the ripe old age of 80 approaches, even with the most healthy, but that there can be even a possibility of this old lady reaching another birthday is a source of wonder to all her friends, and a cause of very natural pride to her medical attendant.

The case is absolutely unique, as far as I know, in the history of medicine, and stands in every way unparalleled.

I claim upon the evidence of this case and that of the woman in whom cancer had returned after evisceration of the kidney, as well as the evidence of many other cases, that scirrhous cancer can be acted upon very easily indeed by remedies, and that the effect of the plant remedy, if given in single dose and accurately selected, is to cause an outflow of cancer juice from the malignant mass.

The difficulty in the accomplishment of this rests not so much in the nature of the disease, not so much even in the selection of the indicated remedy, as in the prejudices of the patient as well as of the doctor himself.

Until Hahnemann insisted, as I reiterate that he did, upon a dose of medicine being allowed to expend itself in the system until it had exhausted its energies, no one ever advocated the administration of remedies in single doses, and so far have some of his followers diverged from his teaching, that at the present time we find our principal Journal vieing with the *Lancet* in its denunciation of any such practice. When we add to the prejudices of the patient those of the doctor, it is perfectly evident that it is human nature, more than disease, that stands in the way of progress. Vested interests are, to use a provincialism, " teetotally " opposed to this simple treatment of disease. It is far easier to get the right kind of disease to be treated, and the right remedy for this disease, than it is to obtain a willing and submissive patient.

I have under me a case, in Kilburn, of a poor woman, who, when aged 62, came to me in August, 1896, with a large scirrhus of the right breast, that had come on apparently from a blow four or five years before, and who had been, two months before my seeing her, to the Samaritan Hospital, where removal of the breast was urged upon her. The woman determined not to allow the operation, and for these two months went on getting weaker and thinner every day, and suffering great pain, principally a shooting, stabbing pain from the upper surface of the swelling, where it was attached to the skin, with pain shooting up to the side of the neck and throat.

Under the influence of unit doses of various remedies, given at long intervals, improvement has gone on in every way. She has continued doing her work and earning her livelihood in happiness and comfort, and though the breast becomes at times hard and swollen with large vessels coursing over it, it has never burst, and is now smaller in size than when I first took up the treatment of it, nearly four years ago.

As to the remedies used, the point of interest in the case centres more, a great deal more, in the method of administration than in the selection of particular remedies, and in the superiority of the treatment over that of operation. But of course during this period of now nearly four years, a great many different remedies were given as the symptoms called for, many of them well known ones, such as Atropa Bellad., Ranunculus Bulbosus, Ruta Graveolens, Colchicum autumnale, Laurocerasus, Nerium Oleander and others.

This poor woman (May, 1900) is still alive, and living a

happy and useful life, being actively engaged every day in pursuance of her domestic and other duties. The breast certainly has from time to time threatened to get large, and at times has looked very angry, but on every occasion the arborivital dose has taken away the unfavourable symptoms. On one occasion, particularly, she came with, for her, most unusual depression of spirits, and with the hard and heavy breast rapidly swelling, with shooting pains in it. Three days after taking a dose of Conium Maculatum ✦ A, the breast began going down, the pain had lessened, and when seen about a fortnight afterwards the breast had lessened in size by one-third.

Previously to this I had often admired the power of Conium over inflamed nodules in the breast, but this was the first time I had seen it reduce the size of a decided cancerous mass.

Anyway, in large scirrhus swellings the action of Conium mac. stops short at decided lessening in size, and it will not, on the same case, exert a second time an equally gratifying effect.

In these cases of cancer in the breast, the doses can be repeated at shorter intervals than when the disease settles upon the abdominal viscera ; in both of these breast cases I have been in the habit of prescribing every fortnight, and I defy any patient suffering from a large carcinomatous mass attached to any abdominal organ, to live through the exhibition of the indicated plant-remedy given at intervals as short as that of a fortnight.

The breast cases require an entirely different system of handling from the abdominal cases ; the one requires a prolonged treatment by remedies given in comparatively short intervals, the other, generally speaking, responds to the remedy at once. Exceptions must of course occur in a disease like cancer, the nature of which may so greatly vary, and where necessarily unlooked-for complications may exist. The fact therefore is that the life history of a cancer of the breast subsequently to the imbibition of the indicated dose is quite different from that of a cancer of the internal viscera.

9

I must in this connection refer to the action of a remedy for warty growths that I myself introduced, the Ferrum Picricum. The position will be best understood by a perusal of my article from the *Homœopathic Recorder*, published in the United States, for November, 1898, and which ran thus :—

FERRUM PICRICUM IN WARTY GROWTHS.

In your *Homœopathic Recorder* for August you give an article by A. W. Holcombe, from the *Medical Advance* which begins thus : "Some years ago I saw in one of our journals (name forgotten now) an article in which Ferrum Picricum was recommended for warts."

As, however, I have the honour to have been the first to point out this very valuable and interesting feature of the action of Ferrum Picricum, and as I have written several more or less lengthy paragraphs on the subject during the last fourteen years, I hope you will allow me to add a word or two.

In 1884 I read a paper before the Homœopathic Congress on the Flitwick Natural Mineral Water and some of the newer artificial preparations of iron, in which reference is made to the Ferrum Picricum ; in a paper read at the 1881 Congress I refer to the action of picric acid, and in a paper read at the Congress of 1896 I specially refer to the action on warts of Ferrum Picricum.

In the *Homœopathic World*, June 1, 1887, and in the January number, 1888, I also referred to its applicability to epithelial growths, and besides, if memory serves aright, when permitted to write for the *Monthly Homœopathic Review*—an honour of which I am now deprived—I made more than one reference to the same subject.

So that I really begin to look upon Ferrum Picricum and its action upon warts as a child of my own. And not an illegitimate one either, seeing that it was revealed to me by the holy ceremony of a proving, the pathogenesis consisting of the feeling as though a wart were growing upon the thumb of a patient.

When there are *many* warts on the hands it seems never to fail, but on one occasion I thought it had.

During the spring of 1897 I treated our housemaid, a girl of some 25 summers, for a crowd of warts on both hands ; Ferr. Picr. 3rd dec. was given in repeated doses, then Calcarea Carb. 200 and 30, then Thuj. Occid. locally and internally, but to no purpose. I then, after about three months' treatment, gave Ferrum Picr. 2x, instead of the 3rd, but still no change. The girl then went away for her holiday, and on her return she showed me triumphantly her hands—the warts had all gone ! "Yes," said I, " and the corns on your feet, if you had any, are gone, and you are feeling stronger," to both of which she gleefully replied in the affirmative. The fact was that for some unaccountable reason the influence of the Ferrum Picricum did not tell until she left it off, which she had done during the holiday, having neglected to take the bottle with her. I mention this, as with less confidence in this remedy one might be inclined not to give it a full trial. But it is in lupoid warts, pure and simple, that I anticipate a great future for it.

In my " Serious Diseases Saved from Operation "[1] is a grand case of lupoid growth taking the form of a large wart on the face that turned black and finally disappeared altogether under Ferrum Picricum.

This case is worth reproducing here, seeing that the lady has remained perfectly well since and without the least scar on her cheek.

LUPOID GROWTH ON THE CHEEK.

Mrs. ——, aged 64, has had for four years a lobulated growth on the left cheek, below the eye, of the circumference of a shilling, and which began as a seedy wart; this wart still remains projecting from the lower part of the growth. She has been strongly advised to have it cut out.

On December 28, 1896, I was first consulted, and then

---

[1] London : John Bale & Sons.   1897.

gave Ferrum Picricum, 3rd dec., which was well indicated (*vide* author's paper at Congress of Homœopathic Practitioners, 1896), and in the middle of January she reported a great improvement in every respect. The growth, which used to cause much pain, especially on bending her head forward, was then painless and about half its original size, and her general health had greatly improved.

The medicine, she said, began to work at once, and brought on pain in the muscles of the back of the neck which spread all over the head, being especially severe on the left side and in the region of the growth; this continued for three or four days and then left. The growth is now (February 6) a fourth its original size, black-looking and shrivelled, and evidently dropping off. Reports, February 25—I am quite well now."

LONG-LASTING LUPOID WART.

A lupoid wart, almost the same in size, situation, and appearance as the last, and in a patient of the same age, sex and temperament—dark haired and bilious—came to me in December, 1899.   Here the wart has existed all her life, but has increased during the last year.   The Ferrum Picr. 3x acted at first in much the same way, causing pain in the cerebellum of the same side, and a chipping off of particles of the wart ; then it seemed to cease acting and the patient went to Italy, and returned with the disfigurement unchanged in size.   When I saw it in May, 1900, I had great difficulty in convincing the patient that it looked less vitalised.   This, however, was evidently the case, for on resuming the Ferrum Picr. 3x, and using a lotion of Acid. Picr. 3x Gtt. x—ʒij. locally, it dwindled away to a third of its original size.

In a case where a working man had a large wart on his middle finger, that had become firmly attached to the periosteum of the second phalanx, and where all kinds of local applications had been used ; I directed Ferrum Picricum 3x. to be given, 7 drops diluted, to go over a fortnight, and at the same time cautioned him that in all probability the wart would not go away till two or three weeks after he had finished the medicine. It ultimately went away, not a trace of it was to be seen six weeks after he had taken the medicine.

The sphere of Ferrum Picricum in old standing cancer cases has been with me that of an intermediate remedy, and if given as such in high dilution it is an indispensable help. Among other indications for it are recurring attacks of jaundice, with tendency to disturbed dreams, coated tongue, mushy stools, or constipation : with, in the male, enlarged prostate, and in the female, retroverted womb and pelvic blood stasis

CHAPTER VII

Cancer Symptoms. — Recurring Abscesses, internal. — Enlarged Liver.—Threatened Cancer of the Pylorus.—Uterine Fibroid.— Uterine Fibroid, another case.

AMONGST the internal cancers are to be found many cases the diagnosis of which, as regards malignancy, must necessarily be doubtful. These cases will come under the head of cancer symptoms. In the following case of

RECURRING ABSCESSES IN DIFFERENT PARTS OF THE BODY,

it was thought by previous advisers that a cancerous origin could alone account for the symptoms. This opinion was probably fortified by the fact that both her parents had died of tumour in the stomach. The woman was 64 years of age, a dressmaker, date of case October 31, 1899, out of health for two years, seven children, married thirty-two years.   In March of 1899 went into the West London Hospital with bladder symptoms: was examined for tumour but none found, and during the fortnight in hospital a copious vesical discharge drained from her.

In the following May, an abscess seemed to burst in the ethmoidal cells, for blood and muco-pus poured away from the nose for two days.   She then went to Brighton and got better of this, but on her return diarrhœa with melæna set in, as if something had burst in the bowels ; this was in July.

Since then has got better of these symptoms ; but during the last week has had much pain, as though another internal abscess were forming, in the lower back.

No history of uterine trouble beyond some flooding at the change ; constipation brings on severe uterine bearing-down, and this is her present condition.   Sleep disturbed at night but is very drowsy by day.   Subject to flushes of heat and feverishness with coldness of the extremities, particularly the feet and legs.

Prescription :—Matthiola Annua φ A. In a fortnight she reported great relief from the pain in the back, but the urine was thick with a filmy substance on it ; she felt stronger and better altogether, the bowels were acting naturally, and sleep had returned natural and refreshing.

Again, same dose. At end of second fortnight, she declared herself better in every respect, though still had bearing-down in front and enuresis if bowels were confined. After the last dose, passed a large quantity of water, and of flatus, and again the film appeared on the urine.

Prescription :—Zinc. Phos. : 3x. gr. ii.—ʒiv. ʒii. td. This I gave for the weakness of the memory along with the nephritic irritability which I considered existed, and in a month she returned, after having gone through a great distress of mind that had caused a certain constipation with scantiness and a sedimentary condition of the water. Notwithstanding all this, her general health and strength, memory, nerves and head were all better ; a dose of Matthiola was again given, and I learn from a mutual friend that the patient is now hearty and well five months after treatment.

Matthiola Annua, the common single Stock, is nearly allied to the wild Thapsus Bursa Pastoris, botanically, and like it meets cases due to inspissation of the juices of the body, gall-stones, &c., as well as offensive and irritating discharges coming from the usual (diarrhœa, &c.) or from unusual outlets—abscesses, &c.

Enlarged Liver.

A woman of 62, very pale and delicate looking, had suffered from enlarged liver for five years with attacks of severe sickness, with a history of having had abscesses upon the lungs and upon the liver. The attacks of sickness last about a week and reduce her considerably. Gets them especially in wintry and damp weather, but practically has an attack every five or six weeks. The bowels are regular, with a tendency to blind piles, and the urine is very high-coloured occasionally. The area of hepatic dulness is markedly increased. A dose of Matt-hiola was followed by relief of all these symptoms; and when I saw her four months afterwards (she came only by special request from me) she was wonderfully better, and had not had an attack of sickness all this time.

Here then is a valuable, because a very common cancer symptom, and demands the most earnest investigation.

As is well known to modern scientific investigators, a fact at one time considered the exclusive property of Homœopathy; in every obscure and deep seated disease, we are often obliged to make our diagnosis depend entirely upon the symptoms; and it is to a correspondence between the symptoms of the disease and those of the selected remedy that we look for the dispersal of the malady. So that we have often to be guided by the symptoms both for diagnosis and for treatment.

I have shown how the symptoms of Ornithogalum Umbellat. start from the pylorus, and that even in an established and well proved case of cancer of this part, it effected a brilliant and unmistakable cure.

The next case has been treated recently, but it well deserves the heading I have placed upon it.

THREATENED CANCER OF THE PYLORUS.

A gentleman aged 52, who had suffered for five years from attacks of painful indigestion came to me early in April of this year (1900).

The attacks begin by a dull aching in the pit of the chest as from flatus, with painful efforts to bring it up, followed by jaundice.   In the May of 1897 had a particularly severe attack, and again in February of 1899.   The attacks hitherto have lasted about a week.

Four days ago a very bad attack began and is now getting worse; last night the pain was more severe than he ever remembers, though somewhat relieved by Gelseminum, feels chilly and as if a sick headache were coming on ; urine high-coloured, bowels active.

Local examination revealed a distended stomach with

decided dulness on percussion and slight prominence over the pylorus. Ornithogalum Umb. φ A. was given, and Carbo. Anim. 6 x 2 grs. every fourth hour if in pain.

In nine days reports: The threatened sick headache went on unchecked, and has since had a general feeling of indigestion, though is otherwise much better; urine clearer, appetite better, bowels more confined and paler. Ornith. Umb. φ A. again. Five weeks after reports himself quite well, free from any pain.

He reports, too, that whereas before the last dose he used to have to lie down on his back after every meal to prevent gastric pain, he can now dispense with any such precaution.

To me the result is the more satisfactory as I had succeeded with arborivital doses in completely relieving the excruciating agony that this patient's wife had suffered from when dying of cancer combined with extensive dropsy.

Uterine Fibroid.

Owing to the accidental destruction of a Case-book, my early notes of the following were lost. Hence the substitution of the patient's own testimony.

" First came under (arborivital) treatment February 19, 1898, for advanced stage of fibrous tumour. Had previously been examined, a fortnight before, by a lady doctor on the staff of the Women's Hospital, Euston Road, who stated that operation was not immediately necessary, but who, in answer to a question as to whether this could be avoided eventually by medicine, declared that this was impossible.

" The first treatment (unit dose) on the above date seemed to give immediate relief. The second (same remedy, R. T. C.), about a fortnight afterwards caused uneasiness and pain, with so much puffiness for about ten days that it was difficult to wear one's ordinary clothes.

" Since then, for about two years and a half I have followed the treatment with various effects, at intervals of from four to five weeks to two months, sometimes with slight pain, sometimes with entire freedom from any inconvenience whatever. After the dose of last February (1900), and again yesterday (May 18), with almost entire feeling of relief from the sensation of pulling on the right side and pain in the lower part of the back, which was almost constant until recently.

"I should mention that when I first came under treatment I was nearly 48, that the change of life had commenced very early, nearly eight years previously, about which time my trouble first made itself evident, causing much uneasiness and anxiety of mind as the pressure brought about trouble with the bladder and kidneys.

"All this of late has almost disappeared, and I am now able to fulfil all my duties as governess in a way which I had not felt equal to for many years, for life was beginning to feel a burden from ill-health and anxiety.

"E. —— F.

"*May* 19, 1900."   " Highgate, N."

10

The interest of this case centres in the fact that the distress attendant upon this tumour, and which consisted of a sense of weight and of pulling and dragging chiefly in the right inguinal region, was relieved instantly by a drop of Helleb. fœtid. given on February 15 ; and that the discomfort kept quite away, the patient not being, as she expressed it, " conscious of anything being wrong" till after the first week in April. Also that while the Helleb. niger, and Viridis failed altogether to relieve her, the fœtidus variety of the plant caused immediate relief.

The tumour which is implanted deep down in the pelvis, bulging more to the left than the right side of the womb, is now smaller and much more movable on pressure than on her first coming under treatment.

In a word, the treatment has enabled this patient, who was practically incapacitated for work to resume her duties s governess with comfort and ease, and with an almost certain prospect of being restored to her former health and strength.

This is a hundred times better than operations, in my opinion, and in that of the patient.

UTERINE FIBROID—ANOTHER CASE.

The next case is given for the same reason in patient's own words, under date June 5, 1900:—

"About three years ago I was feeling very unwell, always tired, with backache and constant grinding pains in the abdomen. I also knew I had lumps there, unusual to most, so went to consult a doctor (Dr. W., of Peterborough), who at once said that I was suffering from fibroid tumours, and that he thought I could undergo an operation in a month's time. I was then taken to another doctor (Dr. M., of Birmingham), who confirmed Dr. W.'s statement, only that I must not undergo any operation, as the chances were nine to ten whether I should pull through, and that I must consider myself an invalid for life, and rest as much as possible. Soon after I was recommended to go and see you, and was under your treatment a little over fifteen months, and during that time and since I feel I have derived benefit. Every one tells me I look very much better, and although I am not able to do any laborious housework, I can do light duties such as dusting, &c., and can superintend generally. I feel it must be your treatment, as I have taken no other prescriptions since I first went to you, and during the past year have taken no medicine.

" It was about first or second week in October, 1897, that I first came to you."

In addition, the patient writes to me at the same time :

" I still continue to feel very well and do not increase in size, in fact, I think sometimes I am slightly smaller, and the fact of having had so many extra people to cater for proves that I am wonderfully well, for I could not have stood the noise and anxiety three years ago."

The remedial agents in this case were chiefly Crocus vernalis and Sativus.

CHAPTER VIII.

Treatment not in Opposition to but a Development of Homœopathy.—Not seeking to oppose any System, but certainly opposed to unnecessary drugging.—The direct curative action ought to be sought for systematically.

IN discussing the views put forward in preceding chapters, friends have often inquired of me my position in regard to Homœopathy. My position is simply this: I act upon and make use of facts that are thoroughly well proved, and that have stood the test of years of experience in the hands of thousands of reliable observers—facts that have failed to obtain recognition from the profession generally in consequence of the natural acerbity of party feeling, such, for example, as the law of similars, the efficacy of the high dilutions, and the prolonged action of the really curative dose—and upon these facts, modified, defined, precisionised, and simplified, I base the system to which I have given the appellation, Arborivital.

The Homœopathic School has, I consider, paid too much attention to the controversial aspect of Hahnemann's revelations and has gone on unceasingly discussing matters that, to my mind at least, are well-proved facts. Advance is, it seems to me, impossible while this controversial attitude is being maintained.

In opposition to this policy I have, in my " Problems of Homœopathy Solved,"[1] put an end to the necessity for further disputation.

At all events, upon the conclusions ˄here arrived at I have brought my practical experience in disease to bear, and the result is, to me at least, in every way encouraging. My work therefore is not, it is evident, as much iconoclastic as evolutionary and developmental : it is by no means meant to interfere with, much less to overthrow, any existing system.

---

[1] London : John Bale & Sons, Gt. Titchfield Street.

It is, however, essentially opposed to the popular prejudice in favour of drug giving, and of continuous and unnecessary dosing, whether by small or by large quantities of medicinal agents.

I hold that between the true direct curative actions of remedies in disease and the food requirements of the body, when more or less healthy, a wide distinction must be drawn. I hold also that the obtainment of this direct curative influence upon disease is a higher, I ought to say a holier, ideal by far than the mere sustainment of the frame by the exhibition of its necessary pabulum, the one being the educated outcome of the physician's observation, the other to a large extent the mechanical industry of the purveyor of food.

The work of the one and the work of the other at times nearly approach, but more often are to be advantageously kept apart.

That an earnest endeavour, aiming at obtaining the direct curative influence of plant-remedies upon disease, ought to be undertaken by the profession at large is, I consider, indisputable.

Whether it will be undertaken in the only way that promises success or not it is for the future to determine; my duty is perfectly clear, and I consider that in issuing this little work I have discharged it.